D1646893

Preface

This book is designed for you, students of Anatomy, as an aid to revision, especially for practical and oral examinations. The answers to most of the questions usually involve more than just a straightforward identification – you may have to think about muscle actions, nerve supplies, courses, surface markings, lymphatic drainage or development – and you will be reminded of the type of anatomical facts that crop up in examinations. We hope that the book will be an interesting and relevant means of self-assessment, giving confident reinforcement of the knowledge you have while, perhaps, indicating areas to which you should devote further study.

Good luck with the Examiners!

The illustrations presented in this text have been taken from the authors' published Wolfe Colour Atlases:

A Colour Atlas of Human Anatomy (1980 and later reprints of the life-size edition; 1985 smaller size paperback edition)

A Colour Atlas of Head and Neck Anatomy (1981)

A Colour Atlas of Foot and Ankle Anatomy (1982)

A Colour Atlas of Applied Anatomy (1984)

Contents

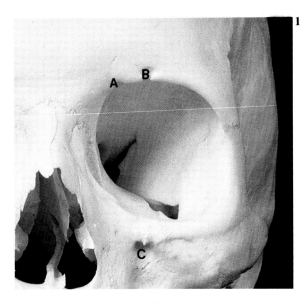

1 Name the notches A and B and their contents.
What is attached above and below C?

2 What muscle fibres lie at A?
What is attached at B?
What forms the bony meatus C?

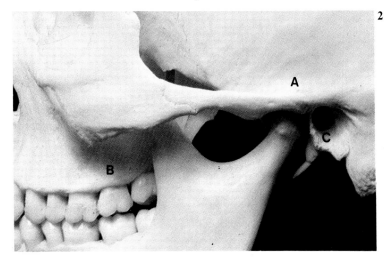

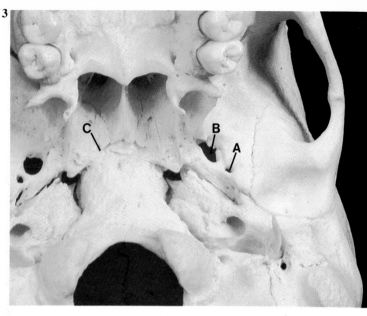

3 Name the foramina A, B and C and their contents.

4 Name the features A, B and C. What is attached to them?

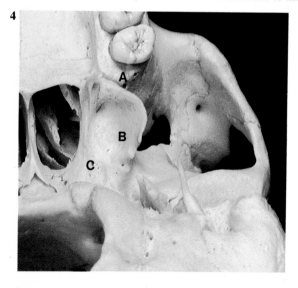

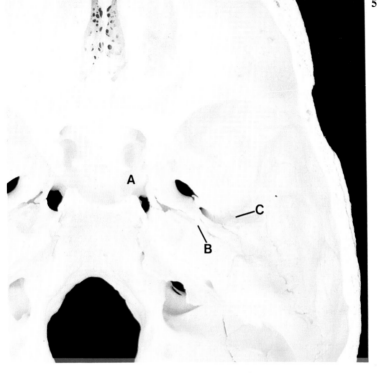

5 What lies in the grooves A, B and C?

6 Name the features A, B and C and their associated structures.

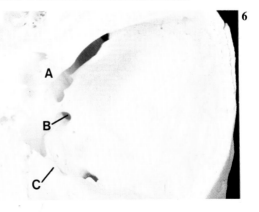

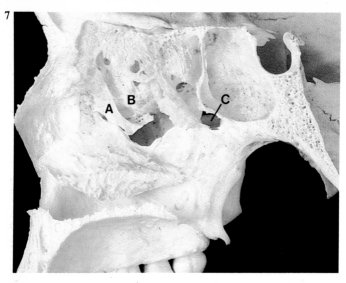

7 Name the features A, B and C and their associated structures.

8 Name the bones A, B and C.

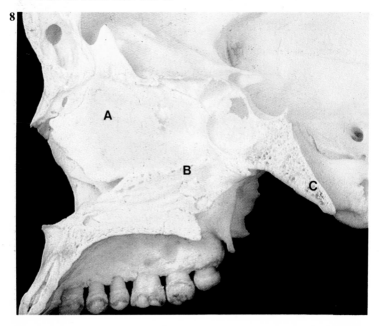

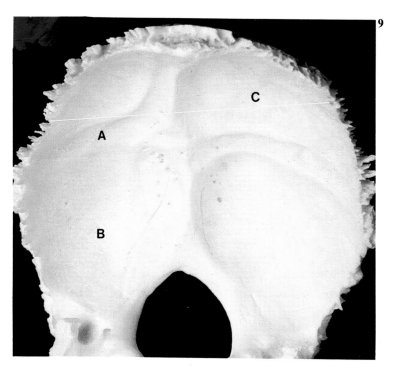

9 What occupies the areas A, B and C?

10 Name the features A, B and C and their associated structures.

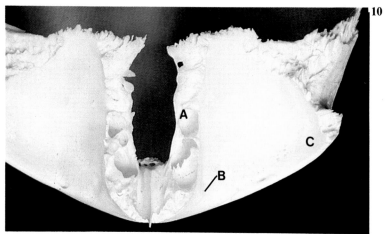

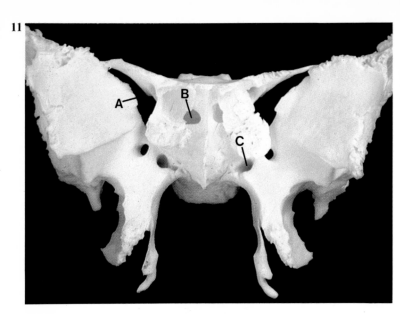

11 What features are interconnected by the spaces A, B and C?

12 Name the features A, B and C and their associated structures.

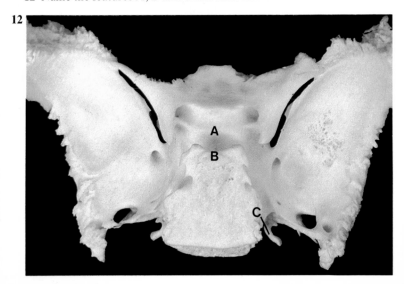

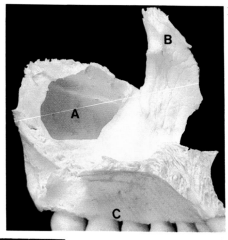

13 In a complete skull, what bones help to make aperture A smaller?
Name the parts B and C.

14 What articulates with the bone edges A, B and C?

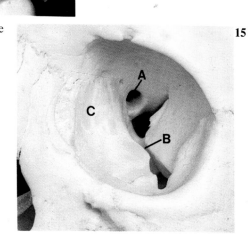

15 Name the features A, B and C and their associated structures.

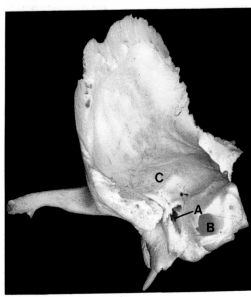

16 Name the features A, B and C.

17 Name the features A, B and C and their associated structures.

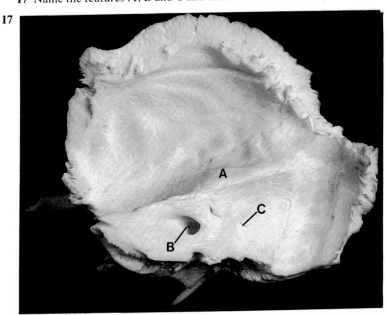

18 Name the features A, B and C and
their associated structures.

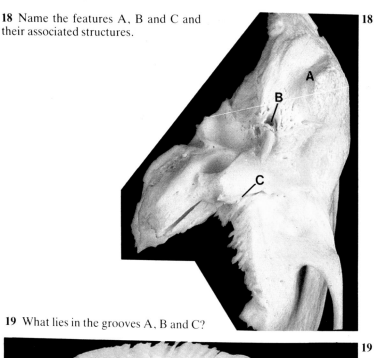

19 What lies in the grooves A, B and C?

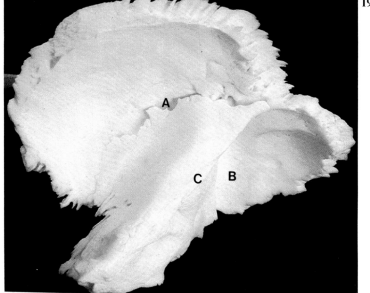

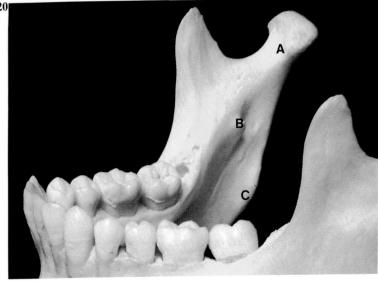

20 What is attached at A, B and C?

21 What is attached at A?
What lies at B and C?

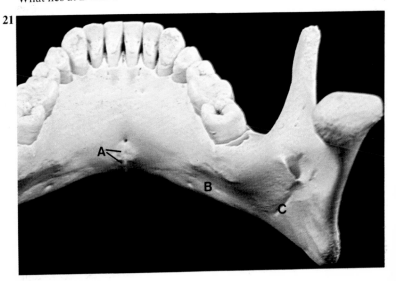

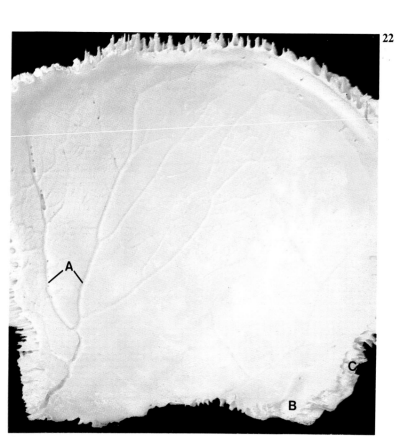

22 What lies in the grooves A and B?
In an intact skull, in which suture does the margin C take part?

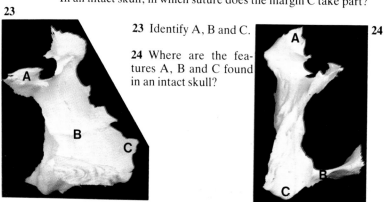

23 Identify A, B and C.

24 Where are the features A, B and C found in an intact skull?

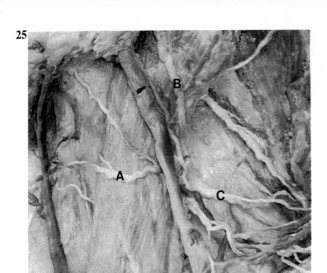

25 What are the root values of A, B and C?

26 How does A begin and end?
Identify B and C and their underlying muscles.

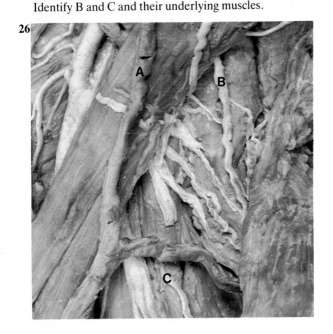

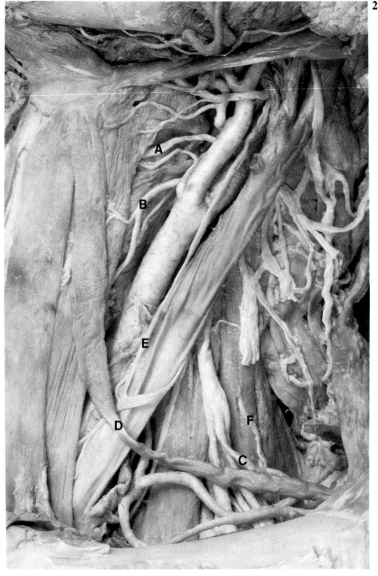

27 Of what are A, B and C the branches?
Identify D, E and F.

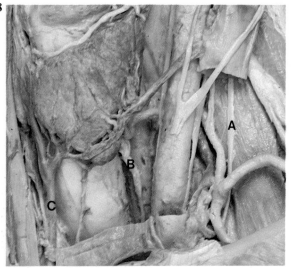

28 Name A and B and items supplied by their motor fibres. To where does C drain?

29 Identify A, B and C.

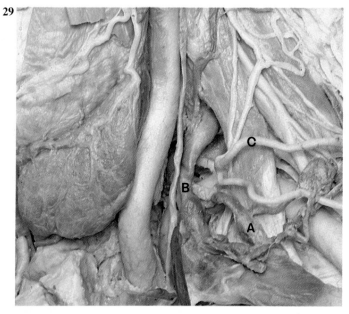

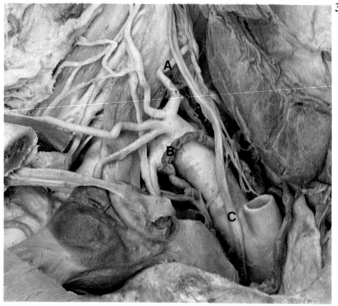

30 Identify A, B and C and comment on their positions.

31 What is the surface marking of A?
Identify B and C.

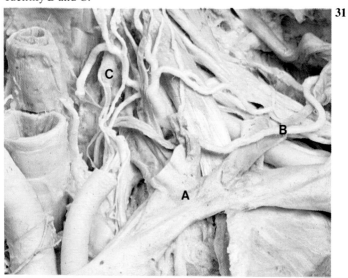

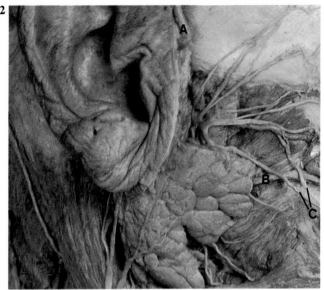

32 What is A and its origin?
Name B and its further course.
Identify C.

33 Identify A, B and C.

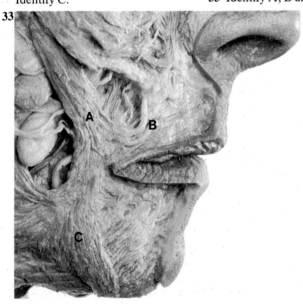

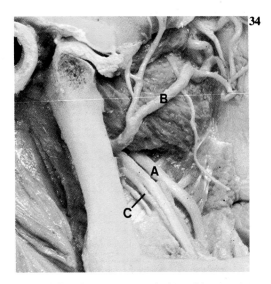

34 Identify A, B and C and comment on their positions.

35 What are the component fibres of A?
What is the origin of B?
Name C and the underlying muscle.

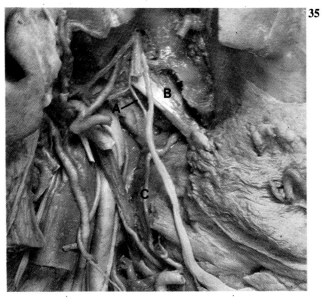

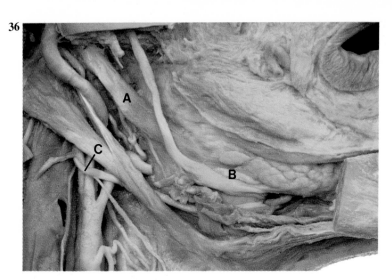

36 What is the origin of A?
Identify B and give its further course.
Name the branches of C seen in this region.

37 What is the identifying feature of A?
How does B get its nerve supply?
What has been removed to display C?

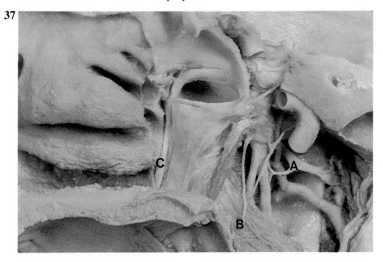

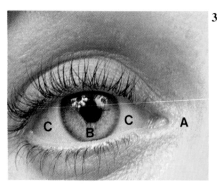

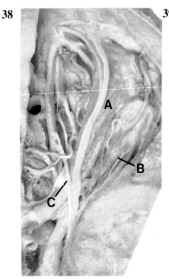

38 What lies deep to A?
What supplies the surface of the eye at
B and C?

39 Comment on the identifying features
of A, B and C.

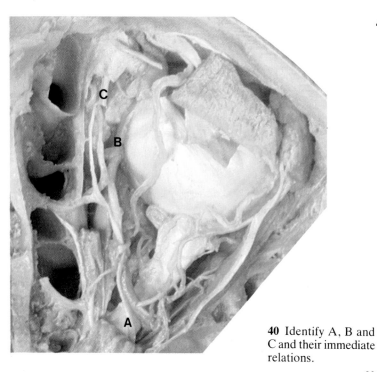

40 Identify A, B and
C and their immediate
relations.

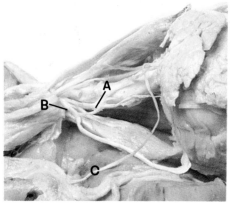

41 What branches run forward from A?
What has B given off proximally?
What fibres run in C?

42 Comment on the identifying features of A, B and C.

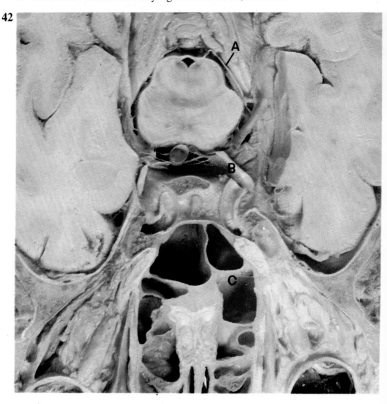

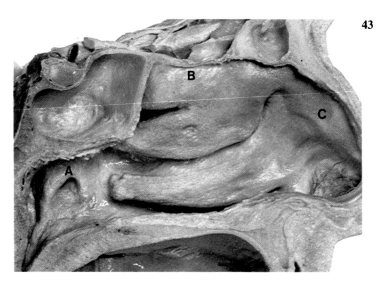

43 What causes the bulge A?
What nerves supply the mucous membrane at B and C?

44 What drains into A?
What do the markers B and C indicate?

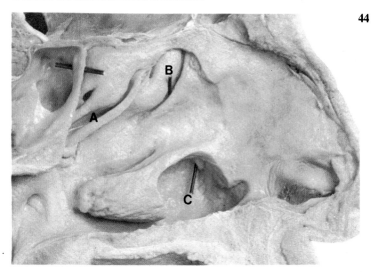

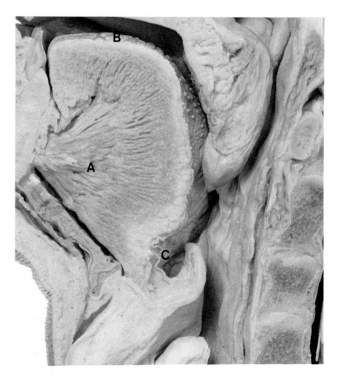

45 Give the nerve supply of A.
Give the sensory nerve supply at B and C.

46 What is the sensory nerve supply at A, B and C?

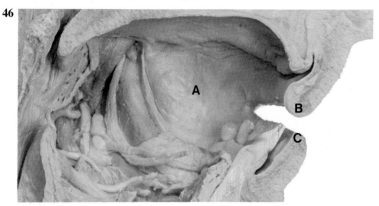

26

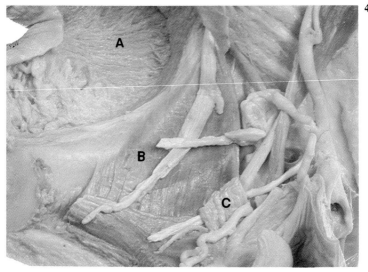

47 What is the nerve supply of A, B and C?

48 Comment on the structure of A.
What is supplied by B and C?

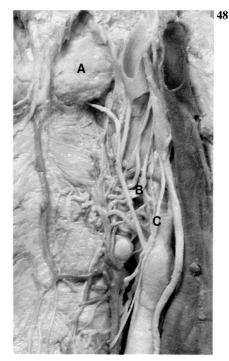

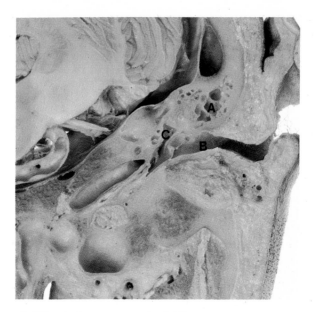

49 What is the nerve supply of A?
How do B and C develop?

50 Comment on the features A, B and C.

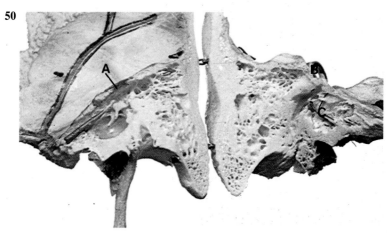

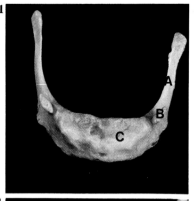

51 How does A develop?
What is attached at B and C?

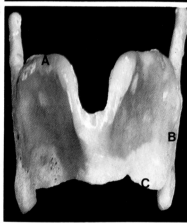

52 What is attached at A?
Give the nerve supply of the
muscles attached at B and C.

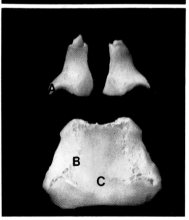

53 What is attached at A, B
and C?

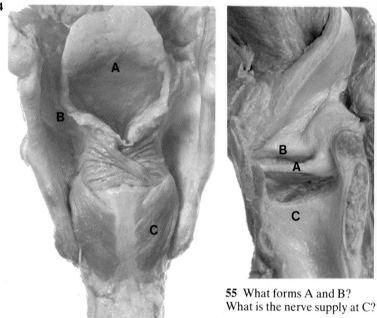

55 What forms A and B?
What is the nerve supply at C?

54 Give the nerve supply of the mucous membrane at A and B.
What is the nerve supply and action of C?

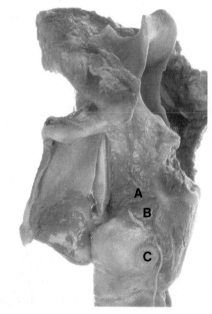

56 What are the actions of A and B?
What is C?

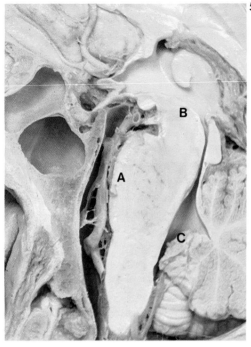

57 What is the blood supply of A, B and C?

58 What is the attachment of A?
Comment on the positions of B and C.

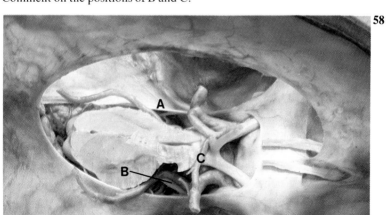

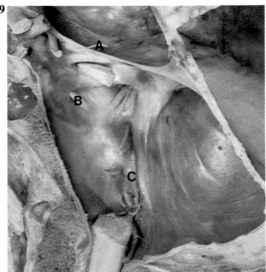

59 What are the origins of A, B and C?

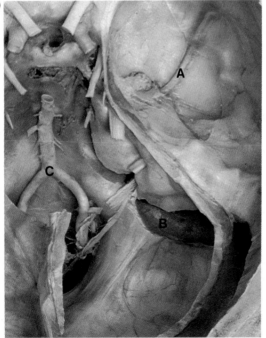

60 Comment on the positions of A, B and C.

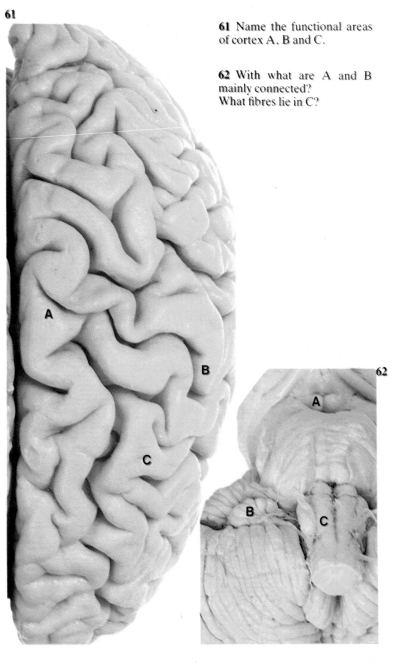

61 Name the functional areas of cortex A, B and C.

62 With what are A and B mainly connected?
What fibres lie in C?

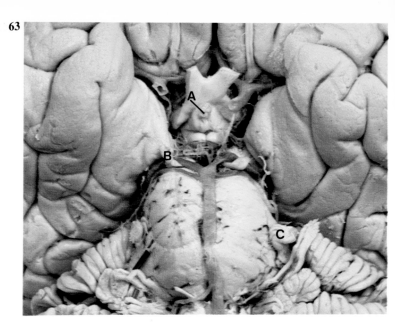

63 Comment on the positions of A, B and C.

64 What is the functional significance of A, B and C?

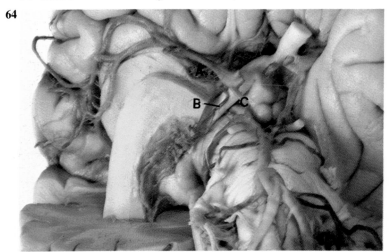

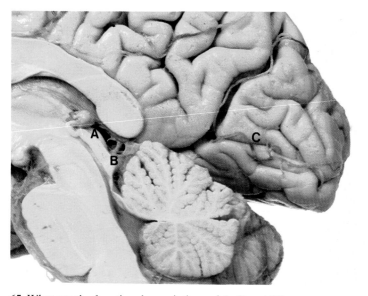

65 What are the functional associations of A, B and C?

66 What are the boundaries of A and B?
What important cells lie at C?

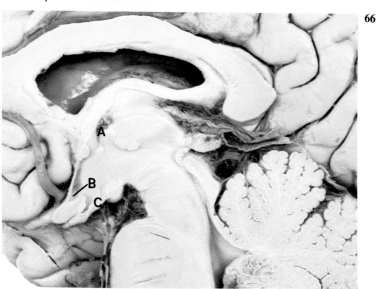

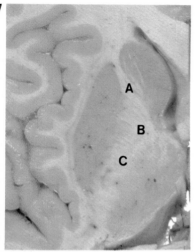

67 What are the principal fibres at A, B and C?

68 Comment on the positions of A, B and C.

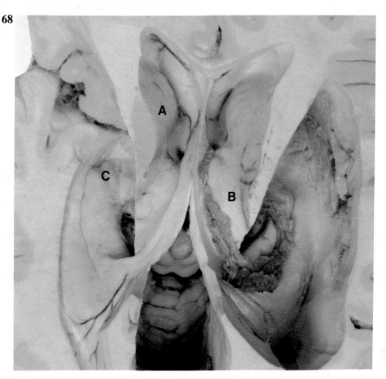

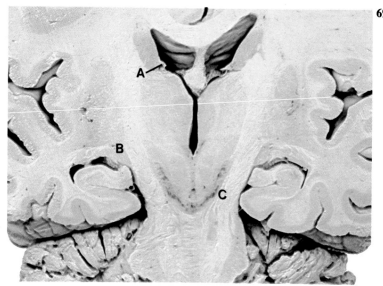

69 Comment on the courses of A, B and C.

70, 71 Comment on the significance of A, B and C.

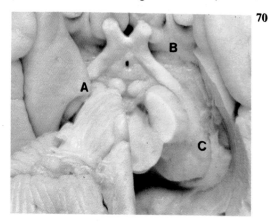

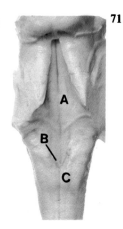

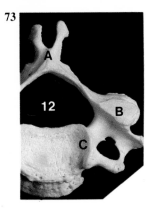

72

72, 73, 74 Give the identifying features A, B and C of these three vertebrae.

75, 76 Which half sacrum is female? What vascular structures lie at A and B?
What neural structures lie at C?

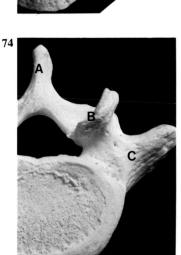

73

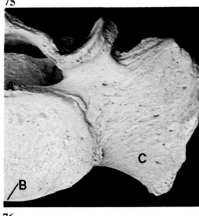

75

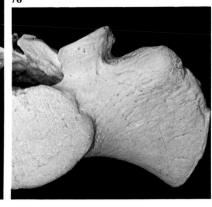

74

76

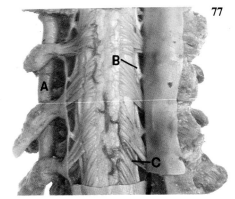

77 Comment on the positions of A, B and C.

78 What are the structures A, B and C?

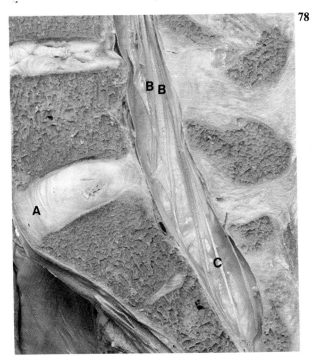

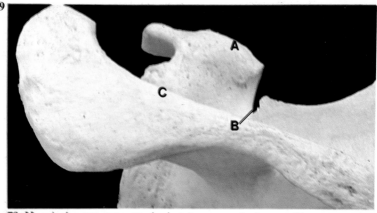

79 How is the structure attached at A commonly damaged?
What lies at B?
How would you test the integrity of the nerve supply of the muscle attached at C?

80 Name the muscles attached at A, B and C and give their nerve supplies.

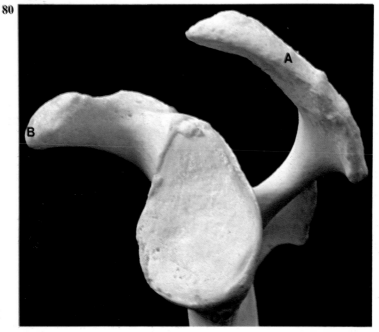

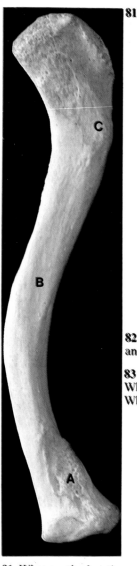

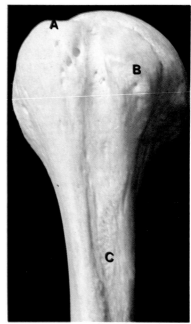

82 Name the muscles attached at A, B and C and give their actions.

83 What is the action of the muscle attached at A? What is B and what is attached to it? What lies at C and what is its origin?

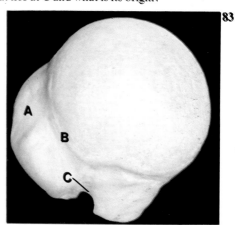

81 What are the functions of the structures attached at A, B and C?

84 How does the muscle attached at A get its nerve supply?
What articulates with B and C?

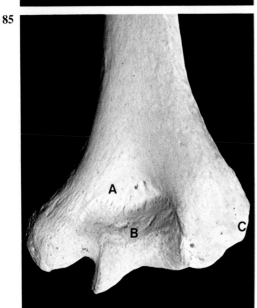

85 What is attached at A and B?
Name two muscles attached at C.

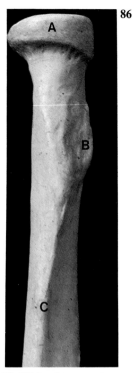

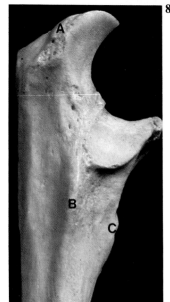

87 What is attached at A, B and C?

86 With what are the structures A, B and C associated?

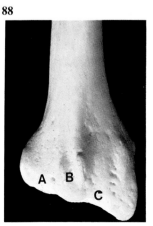

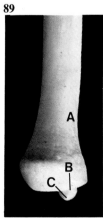

88 What lies in the grooves A, B and C?

89 What is attached at A, B and C?

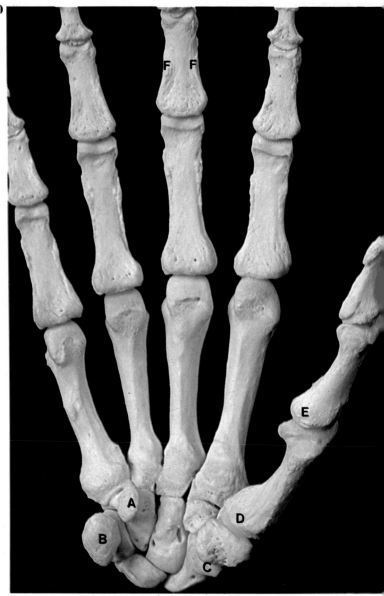

90 What is attached to A–F?

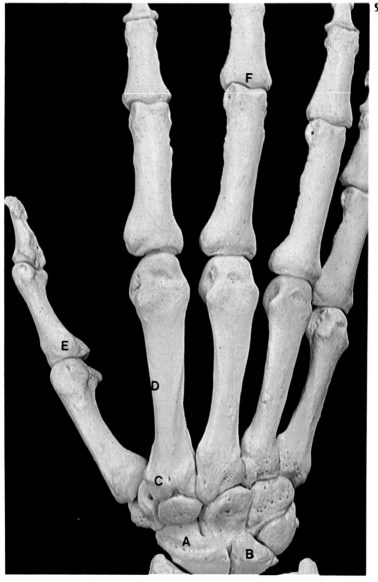

91 What are the commonest injuries to A and B?
What is attached to C–F?

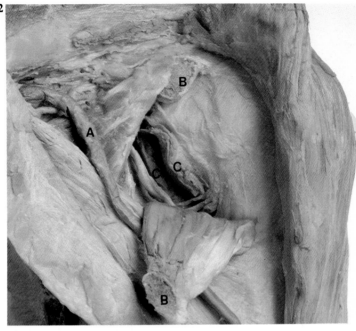

92 Where does A begin?
What has been cut at B and C?

93 What is the nerve supply of A and B?
What are the branches of C?

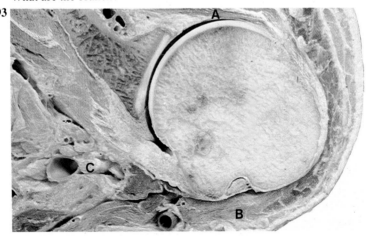

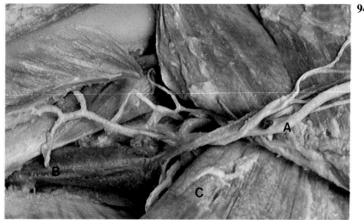

94 What is the origin of A?
How and where does B end?
What are the attachments of C?

95 Give the identifying features of A, B and C.

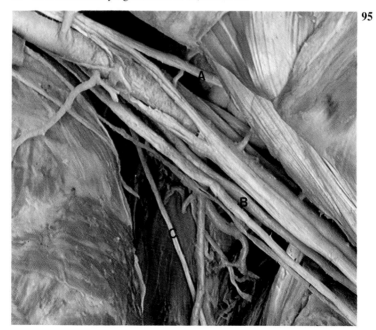

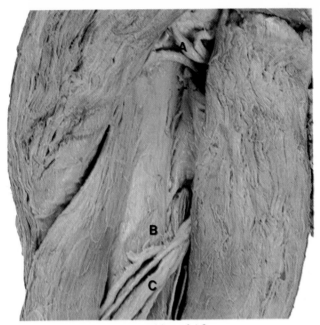

96 What is the surface marking of A?
What is the nerve supply of B?
What is the main effect of injury to C?

97 Identify and comment on the positions of A, B and C.

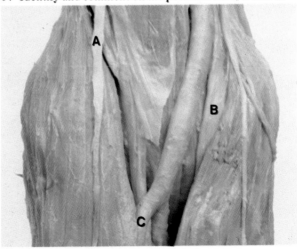

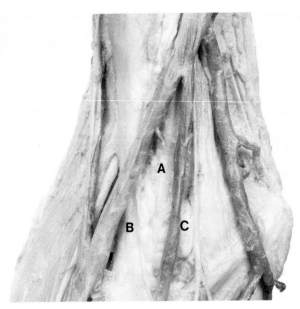

98 What underlies the deep fascia at A, B and C?

99 What lies under the surface at A, B and C?

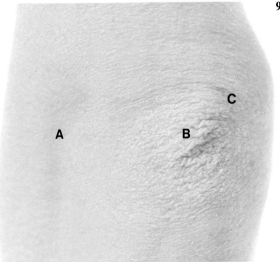

100

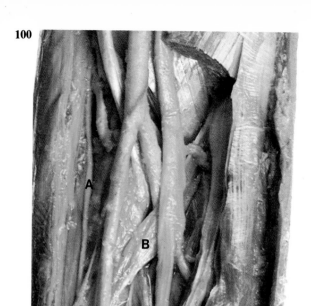

100, 101 Comment on the positions of A, B and C.

101

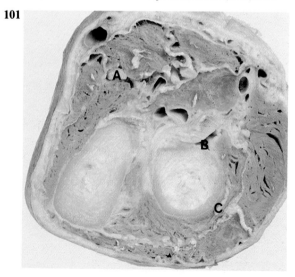

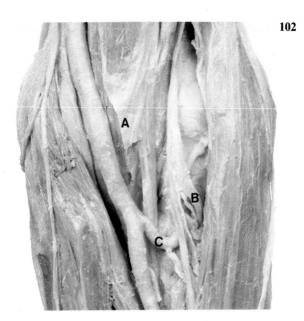

102 What are the further courses of A, B and C?

103 Identify A, B and C and their immediate relations.

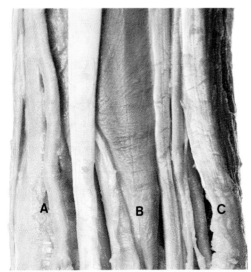

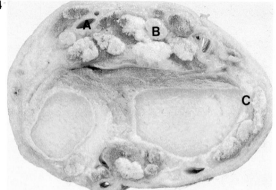

104 Comment on the positions of A, B and C.

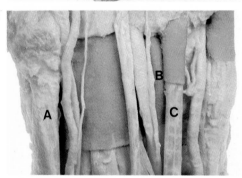

105, 106 Give the origins and nerve supplies of A, B and C.

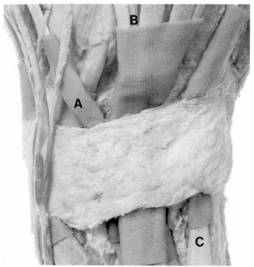

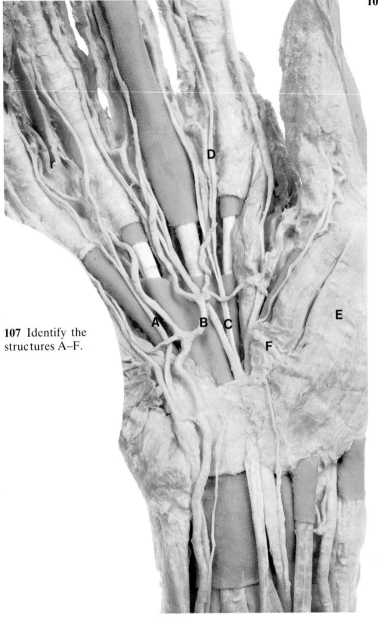

107 Identify the structures A–F.

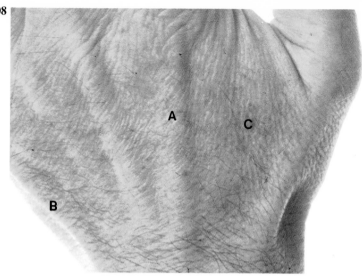

108 What lies under the surface at A, B and C?

109 Identify A, B and C.

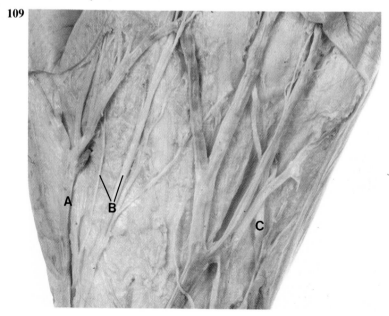

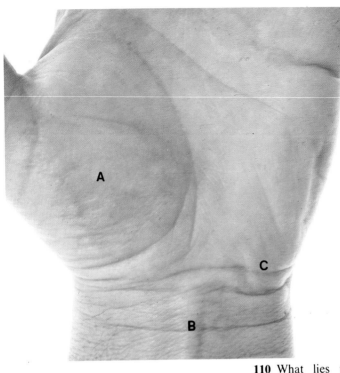

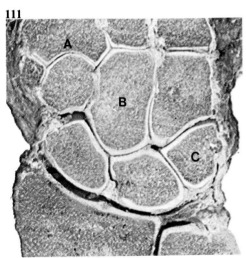

110 What lies under the surface at A, B and C?

111 Identify A, B and C.

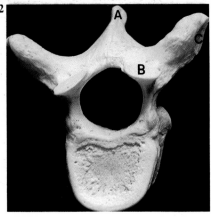

112 How do the features A, B and C help to identify which vertebra this is?

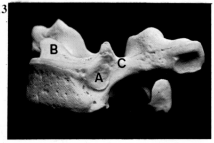

113 How do A and B help to identify this vertebra? What lies above C?

114 Comment on the features A, B and C.

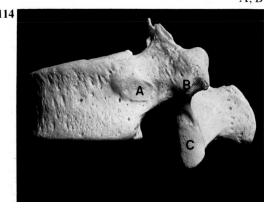

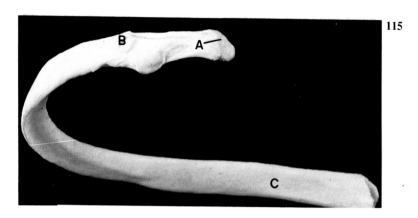

115, 116, 117 What is attached at A. B and C?

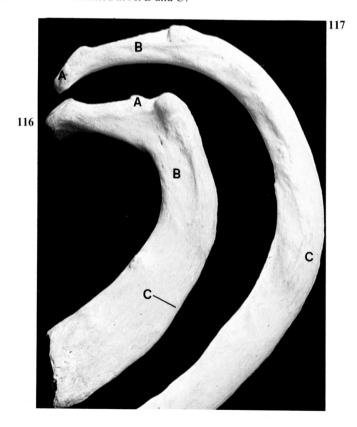

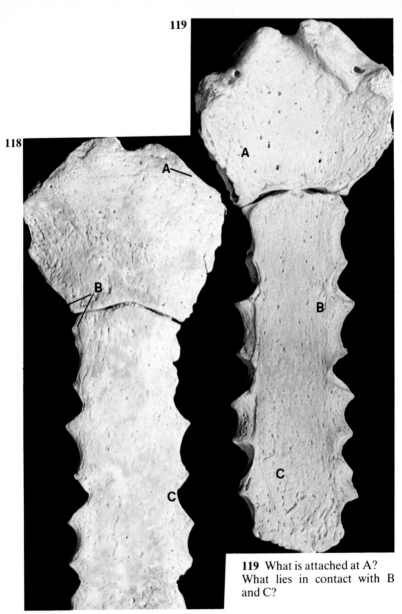

119 What is attached at A? What lies in contact with B and C?

118 What articulates with A, B and C?

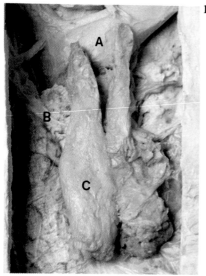

120 How do A and B end?
How does C develop?

121 How does A end?
What is the surface marking of the origin of B and C?

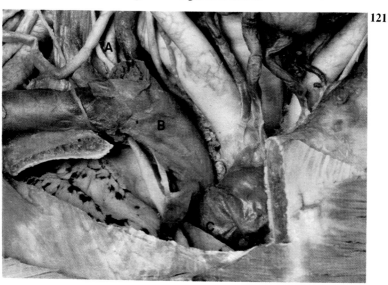

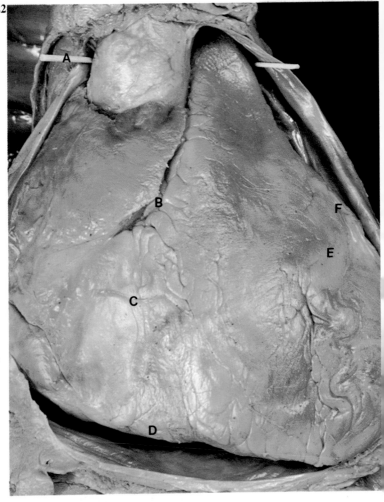

122 What is indicated by the marker A?
What vessels should be exposed on dissection at B–E?
What is the surface marking of the border F?

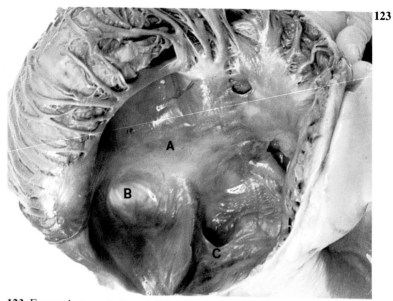

123 From what are A, B and C developed?

124 What is the structure of A?
To what are B and C attached?

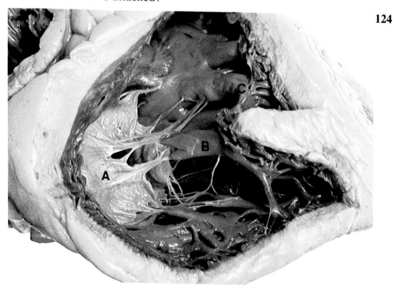

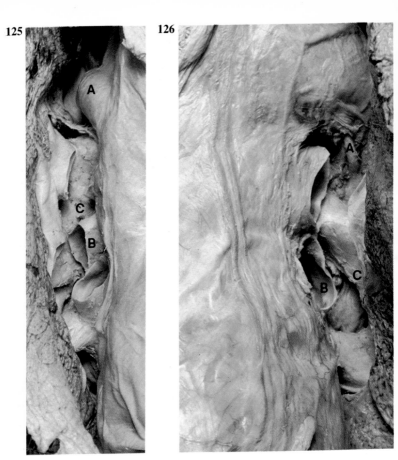

125, 126 Comment on the positions of A, B and C.

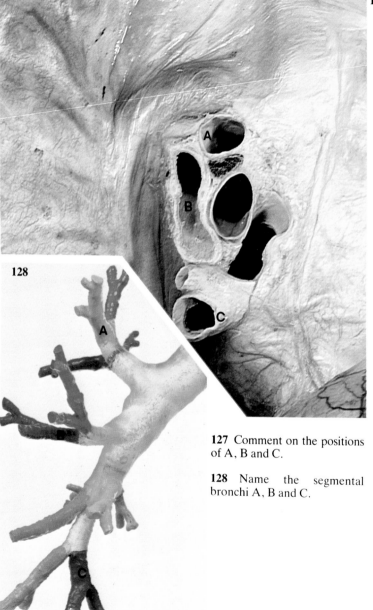

127 Comment on the positions of A, B and C.

128 Name the segmental bronchi A, B and C.

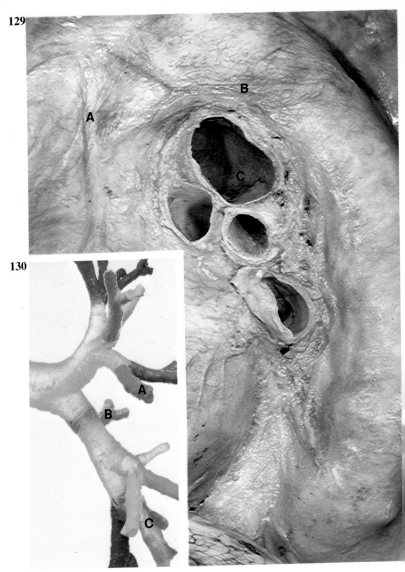

129 Comment on the positions of A. B and C.

130 Name the segmental bronchi A, B and C.

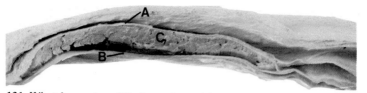

131 What forms A and B above the umbilicus?
What is the nerve supply of C?

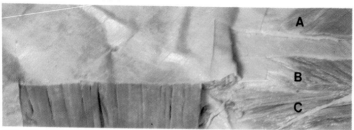

132 Give the nerve supply of A, B and C.

133 Comment on the positions of A, B and C (parts of rectus abdominis removed).

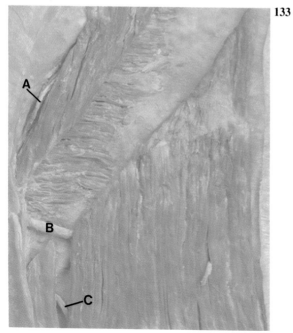

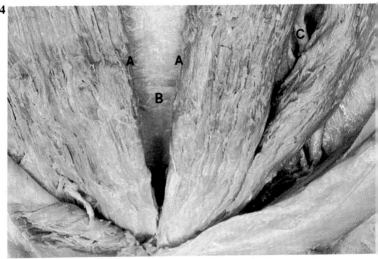

134 In this suprapubic dissection are the borders of A in their normal position?

What must be incised at B to enter the peritoneal cavity?

What is the origin of C?

135 What forms the aperture A and what is its surface marking?

What are the boundaries of the region B and the space C?

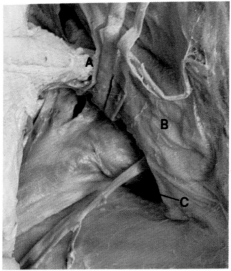

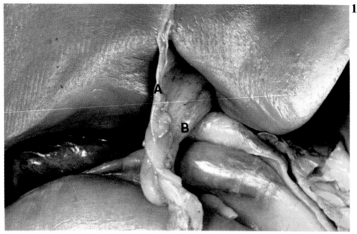

136 From what is A developed and what does it contain at B?
What is the surface marking of C?

137 From what is A developed?
What will dissection at B reveal?
What lies in immediate relation to the finger at C?

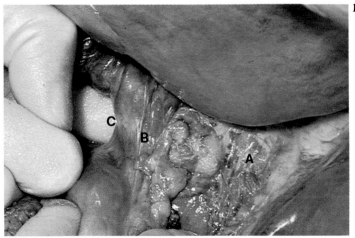

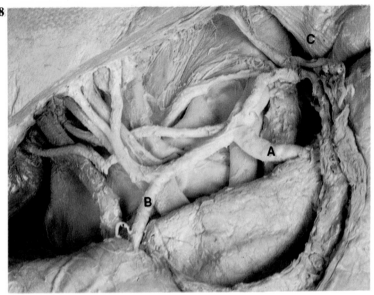

138 What are the normal branches of A and B?
What is the venous drainage at C?

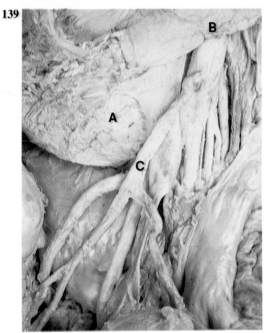

139 From what are A and B developed?
How is peritoneum normally related to C?

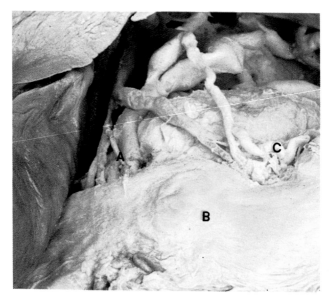

140 To what is A the guide?
What are the main types of epithelial cell underlying B?
With what does C anastomose?

141 Comment on the identifying features of A, B and C.

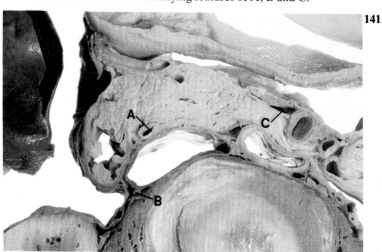

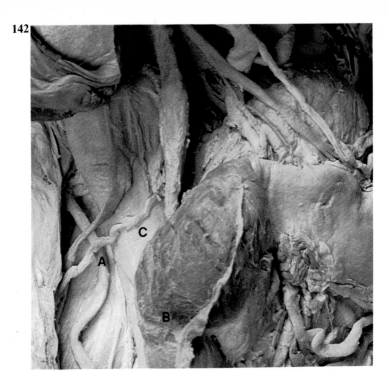

142 Comment on the immediate relations of A, B and C.

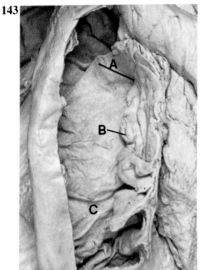

143 What is indicated by the marker A and what is B? What is the blood supply at C?

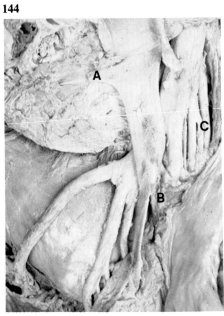

144 Identify A, B and C.

145 Comment on the positions of A, B and C.

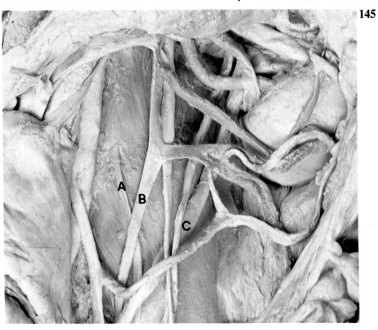

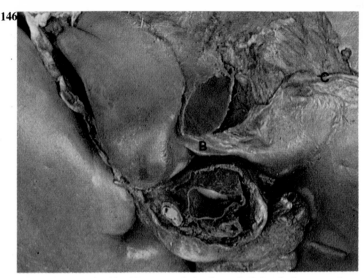

146 What is the significance of A, B and C in their normal position in the body?

147 What lies against the areas A and B?
What lies between the two layers of peritoneum at C?

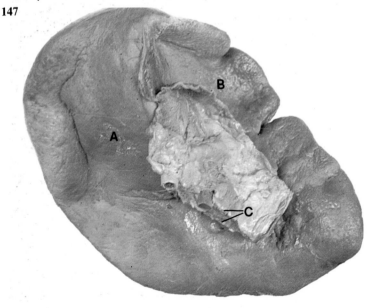

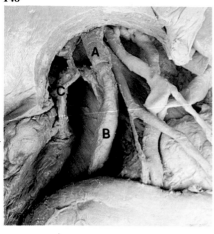

148 What forms A and B? What are the common variations in the origin of C?

149 What is the blood supply of A? How is the peritoneum at B developed? What vessels run in C?

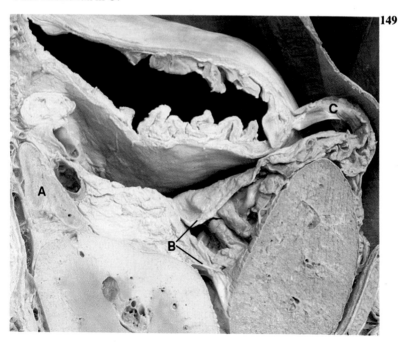

150

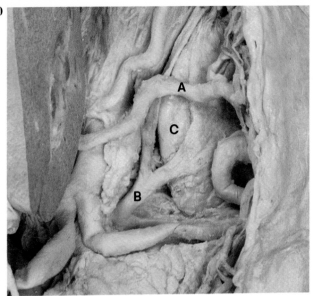

150 What is supplied by A and drained by B?
What normally covers C?

151 Comment on the identifying features of A, B and C.

151

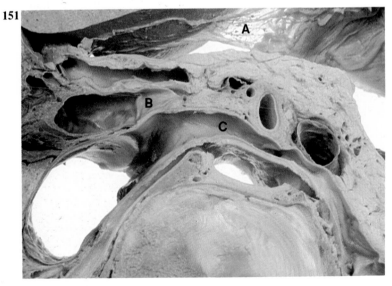

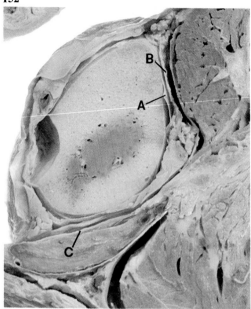

152 Comment on the connective tissue structures A, B and C.

153 What is the surface marking of the region A and structure B?
Is any skin supplied by C?

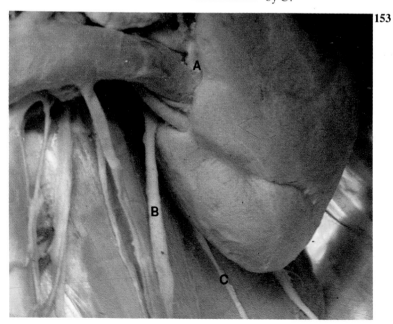

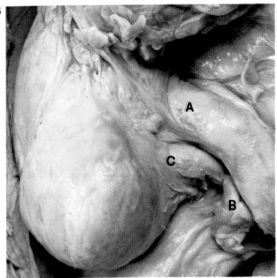

154 What is the blood supply at A and B?
What is the surface marking of C?

155 What part of the peritoneum lies at A and B?
What is C and its origin?

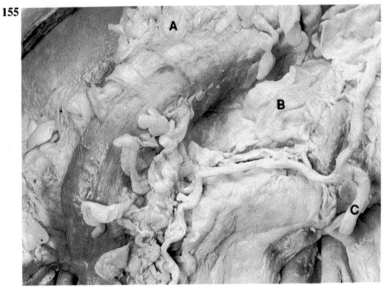

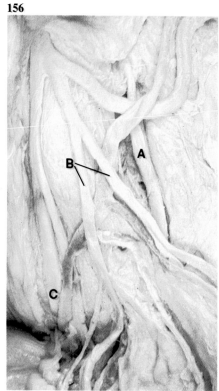

156 Identify A, B and C and their immediate relations.

157 What is the origin of A?
What is the importance of B?
What is the blood supply of C?

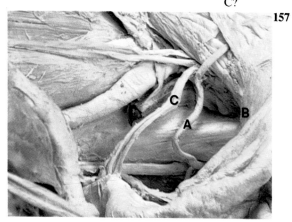

157

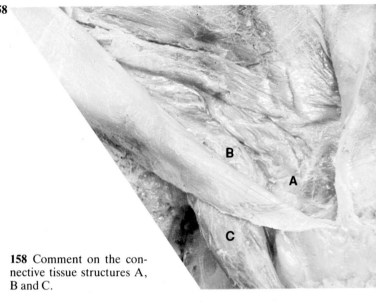

158 Comment on the connective tissue structures A, B and C.

159 What are the developmental origins of A, B and C?

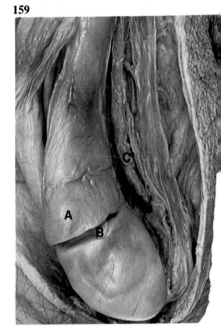

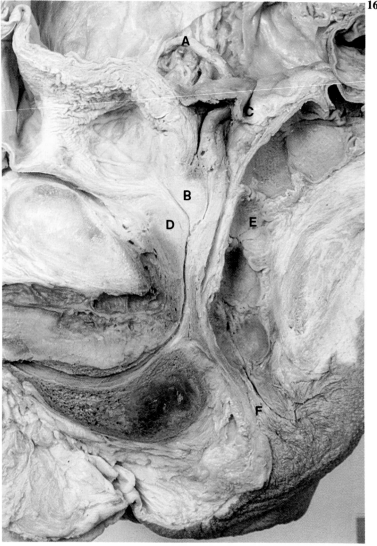

160 Comment on the positions of A, B and C.
What is the lymphatic drainage of D, E and F?

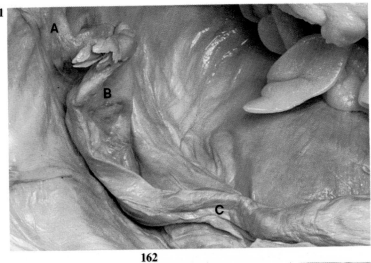

161 What are the peritoneal folds A, B and C?

162 From what do A, B and C develop?

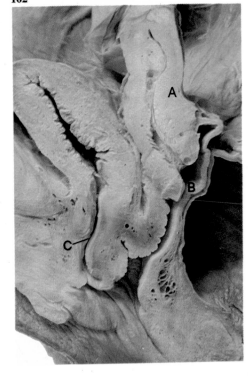

80

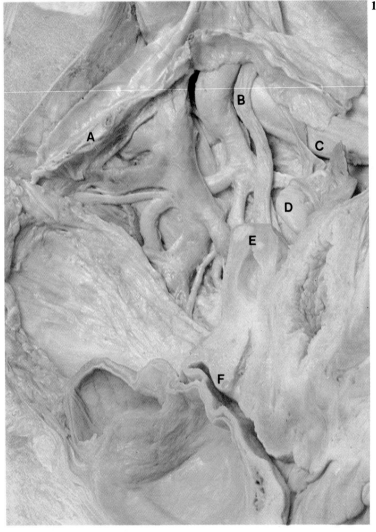

163 Comment on the positions of A, B and C.
What is the lymphatic drainage of D, E and F?

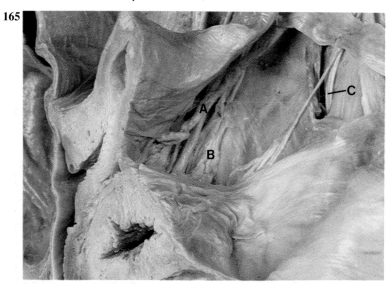

164 Comment on the course of A, B and C.

165 Comment on the positions of A, B and C.

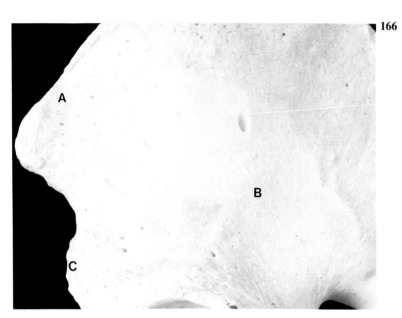

166 Give the nerve supply of the muscles attached at A, B and C.

167 What is attached at A, B and C? Give the nerve supply of muscles.

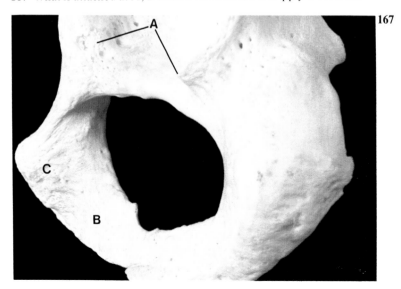

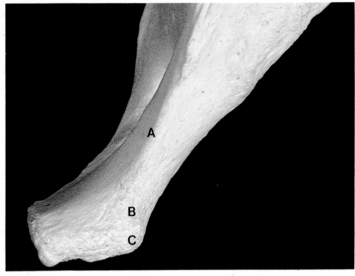

168 What is attached at A, B and C?

169 What is attached to A, B and C? Give the nerve supply of muscles.

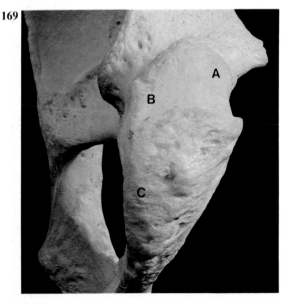

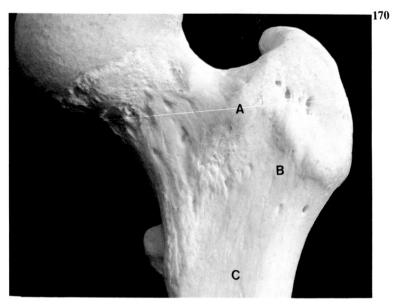

170, 171 What is attached at A, B and C? Give the nerve supply of muscles.

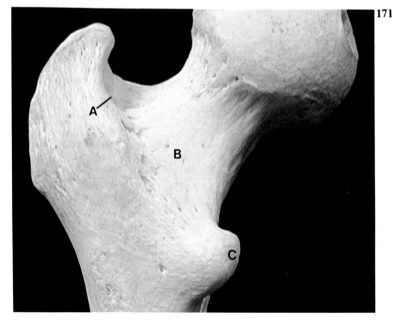

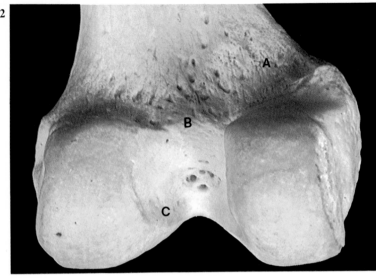

172, 173 What is attached at A, B and C? Give the nerve supply of muscles.

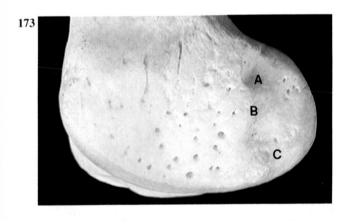

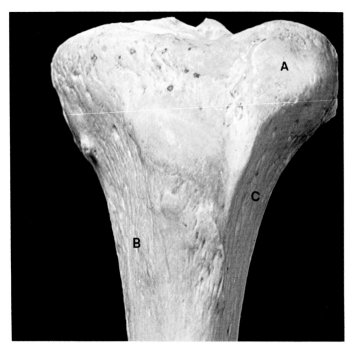

174 What is the action of the structures attached at A, B and C?

175 What is attached at A, B and C?

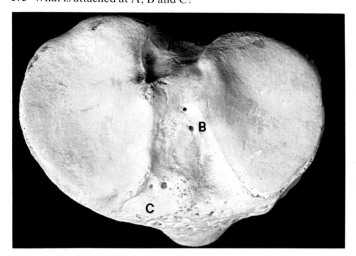

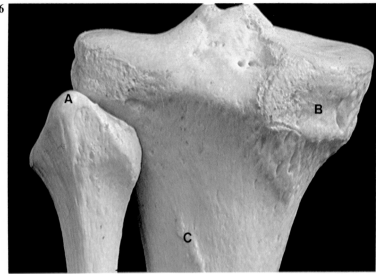

176 Give the nerve supply of the muscles attached at A, B and C.

177 What lies in the grooves A, B and C?

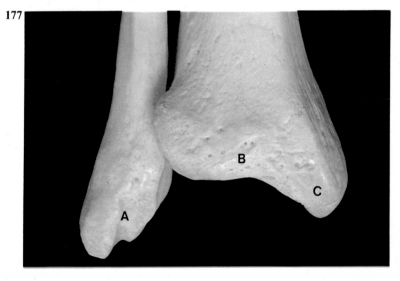

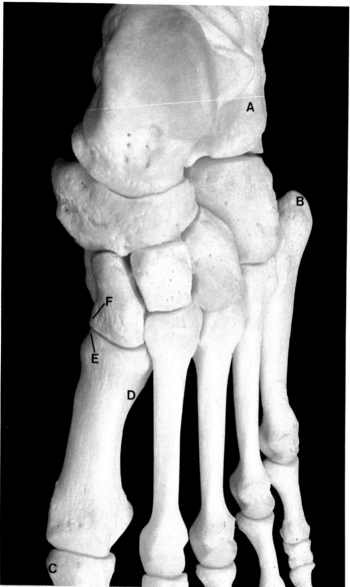

178 Give the nerve supplies of the muscles attached at A–F.

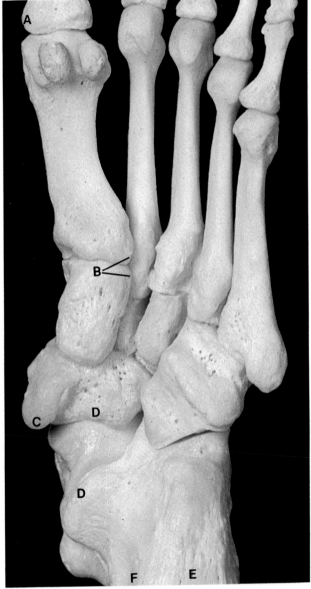

179 What is attached at A–F? Give the nerve supplies of any muscles.

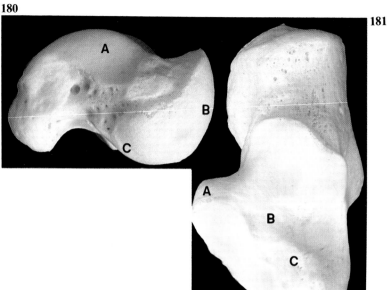

180 What articulates with the areas A, B and C?

181 What is attached at A, B and C?

182 What is attached at A, B and C?

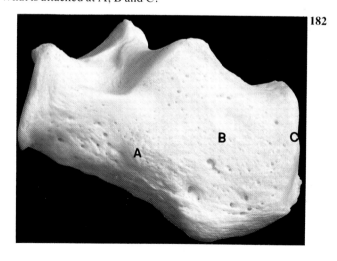

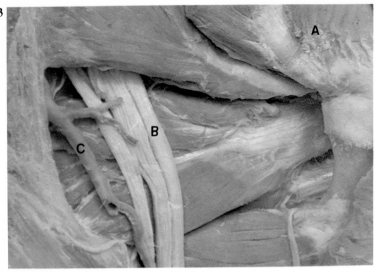

183 Give the nerve supply and action of A.
What are the root values
of B?
What is the origin of C?

184 Comment on A, B
and C.

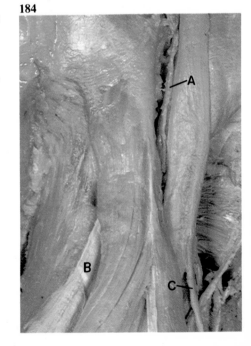

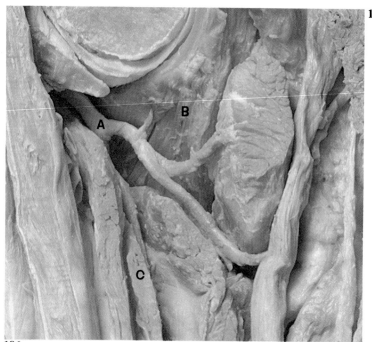

185

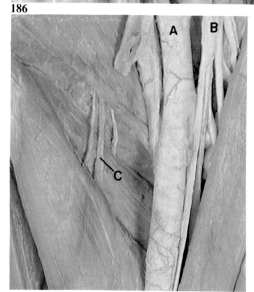

186

185 What is the origin of A?
What is the nerve supply of B and C?

186 What lies behind A and B?
Comment on the position of C.

187 Comment on the positions of A, B and C.

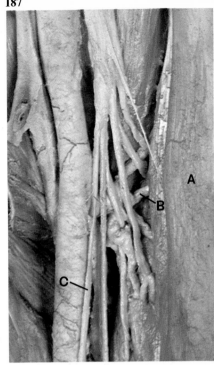

188 What are the attachments and structure of A? What are the lower attachments of B and C?

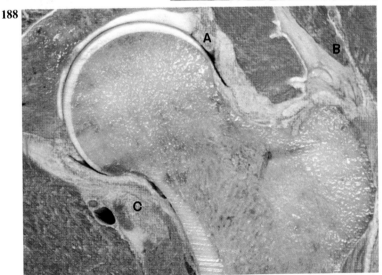

189 What is A?
Where do B and C
end?

189

190 Identify A, B
and C and their im-
mediate relations.

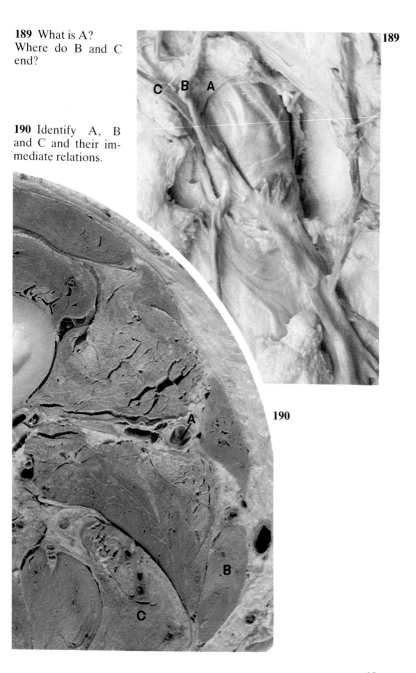

190

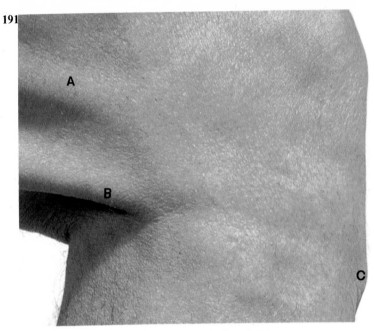

191 What causes the surface features A, B and C?

192 Comment on the identifying features of A, B and C.

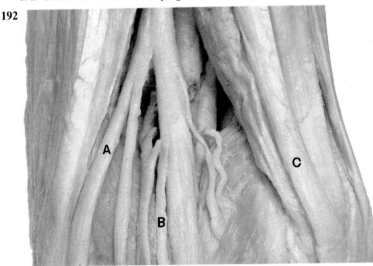

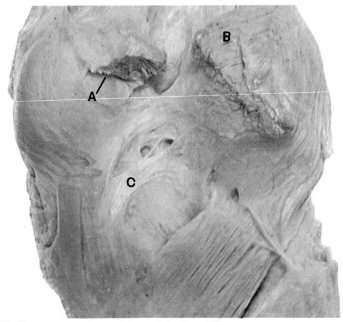

193 Comment on the positions of A, B and C.

194 Comment on the attachments of A, B and C.

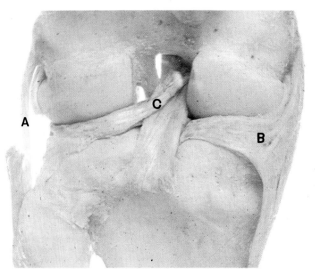

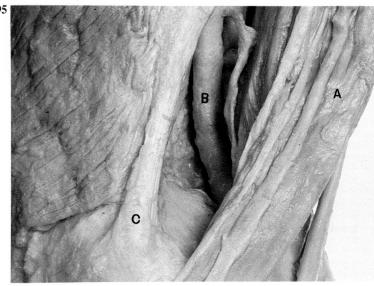

195 Comment on the positions of A, B and C.

196 Identify A, B and C and their immediate relations.

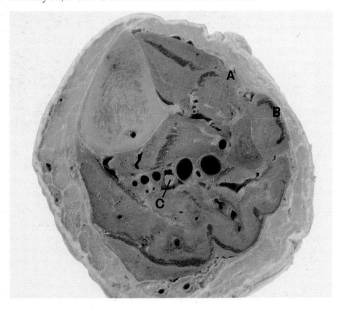

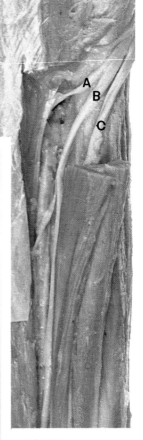

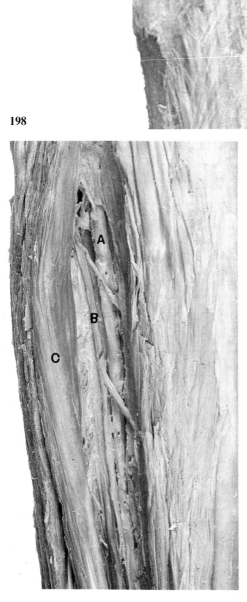

197 What muscles are supplied by A, B and C?

198 How do A, B and C end?

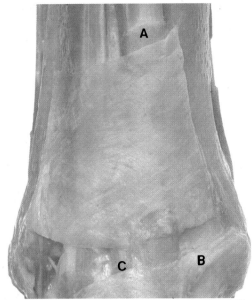

199 Comment on the connective tissue structures A, B and C.

200 Comment on the positions of A, B and C.

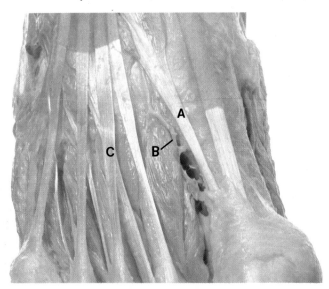

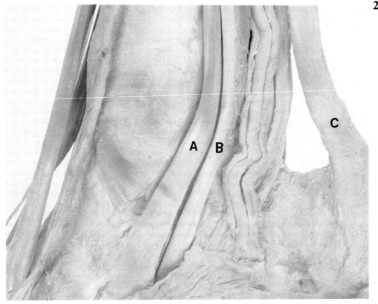

201 What are the actions of A, B and C?

202 What are the lower attachments of A, B and C?

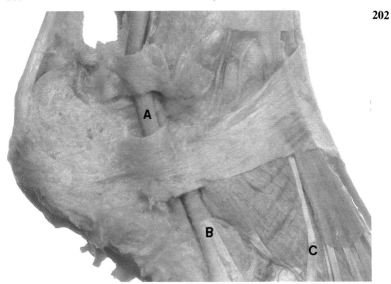

203 How does A end? What is the origin of B and C?

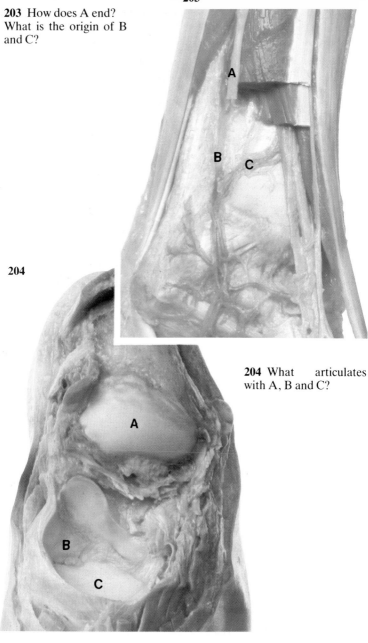

204 What articulates with A, B and C?

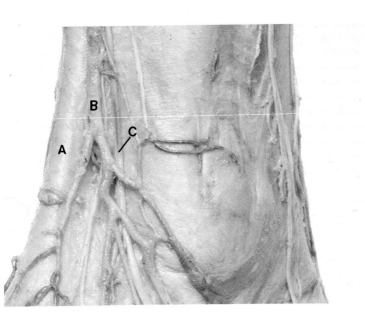

205, 206 Where do A, B and C end?

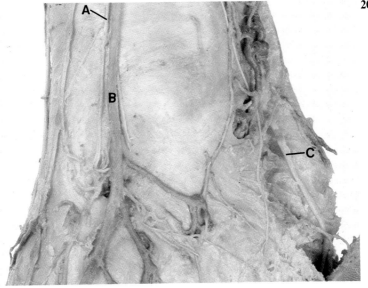

207 What is supplied by A, B and C?

208 Comment on A, B and C.

ANSWERS

1 A Frontal notch (or foramen) for the supratrochlear nerve and vessels.
B Supra-orbital notch (or foramen) for the supra-orbital nerve and vessels.
C Levator labii superioris above the infra-orbital foramen and levator anguli oris below it.

2 A The lowest (horizontal) fibres of temporalis which, by pulling the coronoid process backwards, retract the head of the mandible into the mandibular fossa after wide opening of the mouth.
B Buccinator, level with the three molar teeth (in both jaws).
C The tympanic part of the temporal bone forms most of it but the roof and upper part of its posterior wall are formed by the squamous part.

3 A Foramen spinosum for the middle meningeal vessels (also the meningeal branch of the mandibular nerve).
B Foramen ovale for the mandibular nerve and (usually) the lesser petrosal nerve (also the accessory meningeal artery and emissary veins).
C Palatovaginal canal for the pharyngeal branch of the pterygopalatine ganglion (also the pharyngeal branch of the maxillary artery).

4 A Tuberosity of the maxilla for the lower part of the medial pterygoid.
B Medial surface of the lateral pterygoid plate for the upper part of the medial pterygoid.
C Scaphoid fossa for tensor veli palatini.

5 A Internal carotid artery, in the carotid groove on the side of the body of the sphenoid (in life, within the cavernous sinus).
B Greater petrosal nerve leading from its hiatus in the temporal bone to the foramen lacerum.
C Middle meningeal vessels.

6 A Anterior clinoid process of the lesser wing of the sphenoid, for the attachment of the free border of the tentorium cerebelli. The internal carotid artery passes upwards on the medial side of the process.
B Foramen rotundum in the greater wing of sphenoid for the maxillary nerve.
C Trigeminal impression on the apex of the petrous temporal for the trigeminal ganglion.

7 A Uncinate process of the ethmoid which, when covered by mucous membrane, forms the lower boundary of the semilunar hiatus.
B Ethmoidal bulla formed by a middle ethmoidal air cell.
C Sphenopalatine foramen for the sphenopalatine artery (continuation of the maxillary) and the nasopalatine and posterior superior nasal nerves.

8 A Perpendicular plate of the ethmoid.
B Vomer.
C Basilar part of the occipital (basi-occiput).

9 Internal surface of the occipital bone.
A Right transverse sinus in its groove.
B Right cerebellar hemisphere in the right cerebellar fossa.
C Left occipital lobe in the left cerebral fossa.

10 Frontal bone from below.
A Medial area of the orbital part forming the roof of the ethmoidal air cells.
B Trochlear fovea or tubercle for the trochlea of the superior oblique.
C Lacrimal fossa for the lacrimal gland.

11 Sphenoid bone from the front.
A Superior orbital fissure connecting the middle cranial fossa with the orbit.
B Aperture in the sphenoidal sinus opening into the spheno-ethmoidal recess.
C Pterygoid canal connecting the foramen lacerum with the pterygopalatine fossa.

12 Sphenoid bone from above and behind.
A Tuberculum sellae with the prechiasmatic groove in front and the pituitary fossa behind.
B Dorsum sellae with the posterior clinoid processes at either side.
C Pterygoid hamulus (at the lower end of the medial pterygoid plate), around which hooks the tendon of tensor veli palatini.

13 Left maxilla from the medial side.
A Ethmoid and lacrimal bones, the inferior concha and the palatine.
B Frontal process.
C Alveolar process.

14 Left maxilla from the lateral side.
A Nasal bone.
B Right maxilla.
C Zygomatic bone.

15 Left orbit from the front and slightly laterally.
A Optic canal for the optic nerve and ophthalmic artery.
B Inferior orbital fissure containing the maxillary and zygomatic nerves, orbital branches of the pterygopalatine ganglion, infra-orbital vessels and inferior ophthalmic veins.
C Lamina papyracea of the ethmoid labyrinth.

16 Right temporal bone from the front.
A Semicanal for the auditory tube with the semicanal for tensor tympani above it.
B Carotid canal opening in the intact skull into the back of the foramen lacerum.
C Tegmen tympani of the petrous part forming the roof of the middle ear.

17 Right temporal bone from the medial side.
A Arcuate eminence formed by the anterior (superior) semicircular canal.
B Internal acoustic meatus transmitting the facial and vestibulocochlear nerves and the labyrinthine artery.
C External opening of the aqueduct of the vestibule, a blind-ending sac communicating with the utricle and saccule of the vestibular part of the membranous labyrinth.

18 A Groove for attachment of the posterior belly of digastric at the medial side of the mastoid process.
B Stylomastoid foramen for the facial nerve (also the stylomastoid branch of the posterior auricular artery).
C Petrotympanic fissure for the chorda tympani (also the anterior ligament of the malleus and the anterior tympanic branch of the maxillary artery).

19 A Petrosquamous sinus, in an unusually large petrosquamous fissure.
B Sigmoid sinus.
C Superior petrosal sinus.

20 A Part of the lateral pterygoid tendon, to the pterygoid fovea. The remainder attaches to the joint capsule and through it to the articular disc.
B Sphenomandibular ligament, to the lingula.
C Medial pterygoid, to the inner surface of the angle.

21 A Genioglossus to the upper mental spine (genital tubercle) and geniohyoid to the lower spine.
B Submandibular gland in the submandibular fossa.
C Nerve to mylohyoid in the mylohyoid groove.

22 Inner surface of the right parietal bone.
A Frontal branches of the middle meningeal vessels.
B Sigmoid sinus, indicating the postero-inferior angle of the bone.
C Lambdoid suture with the occipital bone.

23 Medial surface of the left palatine bone.
A Sphenoidal process forming the posterior boundary of the sphenopalatine notch.
B Conchal crest for articulation with the inferior concha.
C Maxillary process, to overlap part of the maxillary hiatus.

24 Posterior view of the left palatine bone.
A Orbital process, forming the most posterior part of the floor of the orbit and the anterior boundary of the sphenopalatine foramen.
B Horizontal plate, forming the posterior part of the hard palate.
C Pyramidal process, filling in the V-shaped gap between the lower ends of the two pterygoid plates and articulating with the tuberosity of the maxilla.

25 A Transverse cervical nerve, C2,3.
B Great auricular nerve, C2,3.
C A cervical branch to trapezius, C3.

26 A External jugular vein, normally formed by the union of the posterior auricular vein and the posterior division of the retromandibular vein, and draining into the subclavian vein.
B Spinal part of the accessory nerve overlying levator scapulae.
C Dorsal scapular nerve emerging from scalenus medius.

27 A Internal laryngeal nerve from the superior laryngeal nerve.
B Superior thyroid artery from the external carotid artery.
C Suprascapular nerve from the upper trunk of the brachial plexus.
D Tendon of omohyoid – a useful guide to the internal jugular vein which lies just behind it.
E Upper root of the ansa cervicalis from the hypoglossal nerve.
F Dorsal scapular nerve (to the rhomboids) emerging from scalenus medius.

28 A Phrenic nerve, the only motor supply to its own half of the diaphragm.
B Recurrent laryngeal nerve, supplying all the intrinsic muscles of the larynx except cricothyroid (external laryngeal nerve).
C Inferior thyroid vein which will drain into the left brachiocephalic vein.

29 A Thoracic duct with its distal end filled with blood because its last valve is proximal to its entry into the subclavian-internal jugular junction. (The internal jugular is here removed.)
B Vertebral vein draining into the subclavian vein.
C Superficial cervical artery from the thyrocervical trunk.

30 A Inferior thyroid artery curling upwards from the thyrocervical trunk and then down behind the lateral lobe of the thyroid gland.
B Right lymphatic trunk crossing the subclavian artery.
C Vagus nerve here labelled adjacent to the cut common carotid artery.

31 A Sternoclavicular joint; union of the subclavian and internal jugular veins to form the left brachiocephalic vein.
B Suprascapular vessels.
C Middle cervical ganglion of the sympathetic trunk.

32 A Superficial temporal artery, a terminal branch of the external carotid (the other is the maxillary).
B Parotid duct, crossing masseter to pierce the buccinator and open into the vestibule of the mouth opposite the crown of the second upper molar tooth.
C Buccal branches of the facial nerve.

33 A Zygomaticus major with the facial vein and artery deep to it.
B Superior labial branch of the facial artery, here piercing orbicularis oris.
C Depressor anguli oris.

34 A Lingual nerve crossing the medial pterygoid in front of the inferior alveolar nerve.
B Maxillary artery crossing the lower head of the lateral pterygoid; it often passes deep to the muscle.
C Inferior alveolar artery entering the mandibular foramen immediately behind the corresponding nerve. The nerve to mylohyoid (from the inferior alveolar) is immediately behind the artery and does not enter the foramen.

35 A Chorda tympani joining the lingual nerve and containing taste fibres for the anterior two-thirds of the tongue and secretomotor fibres for the submandibular and sublingual glands.
B Tensor veli palatini, which arises from the scaphoid fossa, lateral side of the cartilaginous part of the auditory tube and the spine of the sphenoid.
C Ascending palatine artery, from the facial, overlying the superior constrictor.

36 A Styloglossus, arising from the lower end of the styloid process and the upper end of the stylohyoid ligament.
B Submandibular duct; it will pass between the sublingual gland and genioglossus to open in the floor of the mouth at the sublingual papilla.
C Hypoglossal nerve, with the upper root of the ansa cervicalis passing straight down and the nerve to thyrohyoid running downwards and forwards.

37 A Auriculotemporal nerve, showing its loop round the middle meningeal artery.
B Medial pterygoid and its nerve which arises from the trunk of the mandibular nerve.
C Greater palatine nerve, displayed by removing part of the perpendicular plate of the palatine.

38 A Angular vein (beginning of the facial vein), orbicularis oculi, medial palpebral ligament and the lacrimal sac.
B The cornea is supplied by the long and short ciliary nerves.
C The conjunctiva is supplied by the lacrimal, supra-orbital, supratrochlear, infratrochlear and infra-orbital nerves.

39 A Levator palpebrae superioris, with the frontal nerve overlying it and the superior rectus deep to it.
B Lateral rectus with the lacrimal nerve running along its upper border.
C Trochlear nerve, passing forwards from the superior orbital fissure medial to the frontal nerve to enter the orbital surface of the superior oblique.

40 A Nasociliary nerve crossing the optic nerve just behind the ophthalmic artery.
B Medial rectus at the medial side of the orbit below the superior oblique (here cut).
C Tendon of superior oblique (with the muscle removed) entering the trochlea.

41 A Ciliary ganglion, lying lateral to the optic nerve and giving off the short ciliary nerves.
B Nerve to inferior oblique which gives off the parasympathetic (motor) root to the ciliary ganglion.
C Communication between the zygomaticotemporal and lacrimal nerves, containing the secretomotor fibres for the lacrimal gland.

42 A Trochlear nerve, the only cranial nerve to emerge from the dorsal surface of the brain stem.
B Oculomotor nerve entering the roof of the cavernous sinus.
C Posterior ethmoidal air cell, in front of the sphenoidal sinus. Both are medial to the optic nerve.

43 A Tubal elevation, caused by the cartilaginous end of the auditory tube.
B Olfactory nerves, supplying mucous membrane over the superior concha, with cell bodies in the mucous membrane.
C Internal nasal branch of the anterior ethmoidal nerve (from the ophthalmic), with cell bodies in the trigeminal ganglion.

44 A Posterior ethmoidal air cells draining into the superior meatus.
B Opening of the maxillary sinus into the semilunar hiatus of the middle meatus.
C Opening of the nasolacrimal duct into the inferior meatus.

45 A Genioglossus – by the hypoglossal nerve.
B Lingual nerve (ordinary sensation) and chorda tympani (taste).
C Internal laryngeal nerve.

46 A Buccal branch of the mandibular nerve.
B Labial branch of the infra-orbital nerve.
C Mental branch of the inferior alveolar nerve.

47 A Buccinator – facial nerve.
B Mylohyoid – branch of inferior alveolar nerve.
C Hyoglossus – hypoglossal nerve.

48 A Pharyngobasilar fascia, the thickened submucosa of the pharyngeal wall between the upper border of the superior constrictor and the base of skull.
B Pharyngeal branch of the vagus, supplying all the muscles of the pharynx except stylopharyngeus (glossopharyngeal nerve).
C Superior laryngeal branch of the vagus, dividing into the external laryngeal nerve for cricothyroid and the internal laryngeal nerve for the mucous membrane of part of the pharynx and of the larynx above the vocal folds.

49 A Mastoid air cells – tympanic branch of glossopharyngeal nerve.
B External acoustic meatus – from an ectodermal diverticulum of the first pharyngeal cleft.
C Middle ear – from the tubotympanic recess, an endodermal diverticulum from the first pharyngeal pouch.

50 A Epitympanic recess, leading backwards through the aditus to the mastoid antrum and air cells.
B Anterior (superior) semicircular canal, which forms the arcuate eminence in the intact temporal bone.
C Promontory, caused by the first turn of the cochlea.

51 A Greater horn of the hyoid bone – from the cartilage of the third pharyngeal arch.
B Lesser horn – stylohyoid ligament and the middle constrictor.
C Geniohyoid, between mylohyoid in front and genioglossus behind.

52 A Thyrohyoid membrane.
B Inferior constrictor – pharyngeal plexus.
C Cricothyroid – external laryngeal nerve.

53 A Muscular process of arytenoid cartilage – for posterior and lateral crico-arytenoid muscles.
B Lamina of cricoid cartilage – for posterior crico-arytenoid.
C Longitudinal fibres of the oesophagus forming the oesophageal tendon.

54 A Vestibule of larynx – internal laryngeal nerve.
B Piriform fossa – internal laryngeal nerve.
C Posterior crico-arytenoid, the only muscle that can abduct the vocal fold, supplied by the recurrent laryngeal nerve.

55 A Vocal fold (vocal cord) – posterior 40% is the arytenoid cartilage, anterior 60% is the vocal ligament (upper edge of the cricovocal membrane or cricothyroid ligament).
B Vestibular fold (false vocal cord) – lower edge of quadrangular membrane.
C Recurrent laryngeal nerve.

56 A Thyro-arytenoid – adducts the vocal fold.
B Lateral crico-arytenoid – adducts the vocal fold.
C Articular facet on the cricoid cartilage for the cricothyroid joint, with the recurrent laryngeal nerve immediately behind it.

57 A Pons – superior cerebellar, basilar and anterior inferior cerebellar arteries.
B Midbrain – posterior cerebral, superior cerebellar and basilar arteries.
C Choroid plexus of fourth ventricle – posterior inferior cerebellar artery.

58 A Free border of the tentorium cerebelli – attached anteriorly to the anterior clinoid process.
B Oculomotor nerve, passing forward below the posterior cerebral artery.
C Anterior cerebral artery, at this point passing medially from its origin from the internal carotid artery.

59 A Trochlear nerve – from the trochlear nucleus in the midbrain at the level of the inferior colliculus.
B Abducent nerve – from the abducent nucleus in the lower pons.
C Spinal part of the accessory nerve – from anterior horn cells in the upper five or six segments of the cervical part of the spinal cord.

60 A Middle meningeal artery, here on the floor of the middle cranial fossa.
B Sigmoid sinus, here curling forwards to turn down into the jugular foramen.
C Junction of the two vertebral arteries forming the basilar artery.

61 A Motor leg area.
B Sensory face area.
C Frontal eye field.

62 A Mamillary body – fornix and thalamus.
B Flocculus – nodule of cerebellar vermis.
C Pyramid of medulla oblongata – corticospinal fibres.

63 A Upper part of pituitary stalk (infundibulum), behind the optic chiasma.
B Oculomotor nerve, between the posterior cerebral and superior cerebellar arteries.
C Trigeminal nerve, at the junction between the pons and the middle cerebellar peduncle.

64 A Striate branches of the middle cerebral artery, supplying part of the internal capsule.
B Anterior choroidal artery, supplying the choroid plexus of the lateral ventricle and also the optic tract, lateral geniculate body and part of the internal capsule.
C Posterior communicating artery, connecting the carotid and vertebral systems of arteries.

65 A Superior colliculus – associated with visual reflexes.
B Inferior colliculus – associated with auditory reflexes.
C Upper lip of the calcarine sulcus – part of the visual area of the cortex.

66 A Interventricular foramen – fornix and thalamus.
B Supra-optic recess – lamina terminalis and optic chiasma.
C Median eminence – neurosecretory cell bodies that secrete regulatory hormones for the anterior pituitary.

67 A Anterior limb of the internal capsule – frontopontine and thalamocortical fibres.
B Genu – corticonuclear (corticobulbar) fibres.
C Posterior limb – corticospinal and thalamocortical fibres.

68 A Head of the caudate nucleus, here forming the lateral wall of the anterior horn of the lateral ventricle.
B Upper surface of the thalamus, here forming the floor of the body of the lateral ventricle.
C Hippocampus in the floor of the inferior horn of the lateral ventricle.

69 A Thalamostriate vein passing forwards in the groove between the caudate nucleus and thalamus to join the choroidal vein and form the internal cerebral vein.
B Optic tract passing from the optic chiasma to the lateral geniculate body.
C Corticospinal and corticonuclear fibres passing from the midbrain into the pons.

70 A Uncus of the temporal lobe – cortical area for smell.
B Anterior perforated substance – penetrated by striate branches of the anterior and middle cerebral arteries.
C Lateral geniculate body – receiving retinal fibres from the optic tract and sending fibres of the optic radiation to the visual cortex.

71 A Facial colliculus – where fibres of the facial nerve overlie the sixth nerve (abducent) nucleus.
B Vagal trigone overlying the dorsal nucleus of the vagus.
C Gracile tubercle – formed by cells of the gracile nucleus whose fibres form part of the medial lemniscus.

72 A Articular facet of the posterior surface of the anterior arch of the atlas, for articulation with the dens of the axis.
B Flat and rounded inferior articular surface of the lateral mass, for the atlanto-axial joint (the upper articular surface is concave and kidney-shaped).
C Foramen in transverse process, as in all cervical vertebrae.

73 A typical cervical vertebra (fifth).
A Bifid spine.
B Flat superior articular facet, facing backwards and upwards.
C Uncus (posterolateral lip) of the upper surface of the body.

74 Fifth lumbar vertebra.
A Thick spinous process, quadrangular when seen from the side.
B Curved superior articular facet facing medially.
C Thick transverse process joining the side of the body as well as the pedicle – this distinguishes L5 from all other vertebrae.

75 Male
A Internal vertebral venous plexus.
B Median sacral vessels.
C Part of L4 ventral ramus and the whole of L5 ventral ramus uniting to form the lumbosacral trunk, which is the contribution that the lumbar plexus makes to the sacral plexus.

76 Female, having a smaller first sacral body and a relatively larger ala.

77 A Vertebral artery, displayed by removal of most of the vertebral arches.
B Denticulate ligament, with posterior nerve rootlets lying behind them (nearest the camera).
C A radicular artery that has entered through an intervertebral foramen and which anastomoses with posterior spinal vessels.

78 A Fibres of the annulus fibrosus of the fifth lumbar (lumbosacral) disc.
B Dorsal and ventral nerve roots of sacral nerves, forming part of the cauda equina.
C Filum terminale (pia mater) passing from the tip of the conus medullaris of the spinal cord to the coccyx.

79 A Coracoclavicular ligament – torn in dislocation of the acromioclavicular joint.
B Suprascapular nerve.
C Shrug the shoulder (trapezius, supplied by the spinal part of the accessory nerve).

80 A Deltoid – axillary nerve.
B Coracobrachialis – musculocutaneous nerve.
C Long head of triceps – radial nerve.

81 A Costoclavicular ligament, helping to stabilise the sternoclavicular joint.
B Subclavius, unimportant as a functioning muscle but it may help to prevent the ends of a fractured clavicle from damaging the subclavian vein.
C Conoid part of the coracoclavicular ligament, helping to stabilise the acromio-clavicular joint.

82 A Supraspinatus – holds the head of the humerus into the glenoid fossa, and abducts.
B Subscapularis – holds the head of the humerus into the glenoid fossa, and medially rotates.
C Latissimus dorsi – extends, adducts and medially rotates.

83 A Infraspinatus – holds the head of the humerus into the glenoid fossa, and laterally rotates.
B Anatomical neck, here receiving the attachment of the capsule and synovial membrane.
C Long head of biceps, from the supraglenoid tubercle of the scapula.

84 A Extensor carpi radialis longus – from the radial nerve just before the division into superficial and deep (posterior interosseous) branches.
B Capitulum – head of radius.
C Trochlea – medial side of the trochlear notch of the ulna.

85 A Capsule of the elbow joint.
B Synovial membrane.
C Extensor digitorum, extensor carpi ulnaris.

86 A Head of radius – capitulum of humerus, radial notch of ulna, annular ligament.
B Tuberosity – tendon of biceps and bursa.
C Anterior oblique line – attachment of the radial head of flexor digitorum superficialis.

87 A Olecranon – triceps.
B Supinator crest – part of the origin of supinator.
C Tuberosity of ulna – brachialis.

88 A Extensor digitorum and extensor indicis.
B Extensor pollicis longus.
C Extensor carpi radialis brevis.

89 A Pronator quadratus.
B Articular disc, separating the inferior radio-ulnar joint from the wrist joint.
C Ulnar collateral ligament of the wrist joint.

90 A Hook of hamate – pisohamate ligament, flexor retinaculum, flexor digiti minimi brevis, opponens digiti minimi.
B Pisiform – flexor carpi ulnaris, abductor digiti minimi, pisohamate ligament, pisometacarpal ligament, flexor retinaculum, extensor retinaculum.
C Tubercle of scaphoid – flexor retinaculum, abductor pollicis brevis.
D Radial side of base of first metacarpal – abductor pollicis longus.
E Radial side of base of proximal phalanx – flexor and abductor pollicis brevis.
F Sides of shaft of middle phalanx – flexor digitorum superficialis.

91 A Scaphoid – the carpal bone most commonly fractured.
B Lunate – the carpal bone most commonly dislocated.
C Extensor carpi radialis longus.
D First dorsal interosseous.
E Insertion of first dorsal interosseous and adductor pollicis.
F Dorsal digital expansion.

92 A Cephalic vein – begins in the anatomical snuffbox.
B Coracoid process, here turned down with coracobrachialis and the short head of biceps attached.
C Subscapularis, cut to expose the capsule of the shoulder joint.

93 A Infraspinatus – suprascapular nerve.
B Deltoid – axillary nerve.
C Lateral cord of the brachial plexus, giving rise to the lateral pectoral and musculocutaneous nerves and the lateral root of the median nerve.

94 A Pectoral branch of the thoraco-acromial artery, from the second part of the axillary artery.
B Subclavian vein – ending by joining the internal jugular vein to form the brachiocephalic vein.
C Pectoralis minor – from the third, fourth and fifth ribs to the medial side of the coracoid process.

95 A Musculocutaneous nerve arising from the lateral cord and entering coraco-brachialis.
B Ulnar nerve arising from the medial cord and passing down between the axillary artery and axillary vein (here removed) just behind the medial cutaneous nerve of forearm which is slightly smaller than the ulnar nerve and must not be confused with it.
C Thoracodorsal nerve (to latissumus dorsi) from the posterior cord and accompanying the thoracodorsal artery (from the subscapular) on the posterior axillary wall.

96 A Axillary nerve – passing round behind the humerus at a level about 6 cm below the acromion.
B Medial head of triceps – by two branches from the radial nerve.
C Radial nerve – "wrist drop" due to paralysis of the extensor muscles.

97 A Lateral cutaneous nerve of forearm, the continuation of the musculocutaneous nerve, becoming superficial where the muscle fibres of biceps become tendinous.
B Median nerve lying medial to the brachial artery which in turn is medial to the biceps tendon. The nerve is becoming crossed by pronator teres.
C Radial artery becoming overlapped by brachioradialis.

98 A Brachial artery.
B Tendon of biceps.
C Median nerve.

99 A Head of the radius.
B Olecranon and the olecranon bursa.
C Ulnar nerve.

100 A Superficial branch of the radial nerve, displayed by displacing brachioradialis laterally.
B Deep head of pronator teres separating the median nerve and ulnar artery.
C Radial head of flexor digitorum superficialis with the median nerve passing deep to its upper edge.

101 Cross section of left upper forearm, from below.
A Ulnar nerve between flexor digitorum superficialis and flexor digitorum profundus.
B Bursa between the tendon of biceps and the radial tuberosity.
C Posterior interosseous nerve embedded in supinator.

102 A Bicipital aponeurosis (here cut) which should pass obliquely downwards over the brachial artery and median nerve to fuse with the deep fascia.
B Posterior interosseous nerve, which will enter supinator and emerge in the posterior compartment of the forearm to supply extensor muscles.
C Radial recurrent artery, passing upwards on supinator to anastomose with a branch of the profunda brachii artery.

103 A Pronator quadratus with the radial artery overlying it.
B Flexor digitorum superficialis with the median nerve becoming superficial by curling round its radial side.
C Flexor carpi ulnaris, displaced slightly medially to display the ulnar nerve and artery.

104 Cross section of the left lower forearm, from below.
A Ulnar artery, partly overlapped by flexor carpi ulnaris and with the ulnar nerve on its medial side.
B Median nerve, with flexor carpi radialis on lateral side and flexor digitorum superficialis medially.
C Insertion of brachioradialis, crossed by the tendons of abductor pollicis longus and extensor pollicis brevis.

105 A Flexor carpi ulnaris – ulnar head from the posterior border of the ulna and medial margin of the olecranon, and a small humeral head from the common flexor origin (medial epicondyle of the humerus). Supplied by the ulnar nerve.
B Flexor pollicis longus – anterior surface of the radius below the tuberosity, the interosseous membrane, and a small slip from the lateral or medial side of the coronoid process. Supplied by the anterior interosseous branch of the median nerve.
C Flexor carpi radialis – common flexor origin. Supplied by the median nerve.

106 A Extensor pollicis longus – middle of the posterior surface of the ulna (below abductor pollicis longus) and the interosseous membrane. Supplied by the posterior interosseous nerve.
B Extensor indicis – posterior surface of the ulna (below extensor pollicis longus) and the interosseous membrane. Supplied by the posterior interosseous nerve.
C Extensor carpi ulnaris – common extensor origin (lateral epicondyle of the humerus) and the posterior border of the ulna. Supplied by the posterior interosseous nerve.

107 A   A common palmar digital branch of the ulnar nerve.
B   Superficial palmar arch, the continuation of the ulnar artery.
C   A common palmar digital branch of the median nerve.
D   A palmar digital branch of the median nerve.
E   Abductor pollicis brevis lying on the radial side of flexor pollicis brevis.
F   Muscular (recurrent) branch of the median nerve, usually supplying flexor and abductor pollicis brevis and opponens pollicis.

108 A   Extensor digitorum tendon, with extensor indicis tendon on the ulnar side.
B   Double tendon of extensor digiti minimi (this is normal).
C   First dorsal interosseous muscle.

109 A   Cephalic vein.
B   Radial nerve branches.
C   Dorsal branch of the ulnar nerve.

110 A   Flexor pollicis brevis.
B   Palmaris longus tendon, slightly overlapping the median nerve on the radial side of the tendon.
C   Ulnar artery and nerve, lying on the radial side of the pisiform.

111 A   Base of the second metacarpal bone.
B   Capitate bone.
C   Triquetral bone.

112 A   Spinous process not bifid or massive.
B   Superior articular facet is vertical, flat and faces slightly laterally – all thoracic characteristics.
C   Transverse process has an articular facet for the tubercle of a rib – another thoracic characteristic.

113 A   Upper costal facet on the body is completely round.
B   Uncus (posterolateral lip) on a body with costal facets identifies T1 vertebra.
C   Above but not in contact lies the meningeal sheath containing C8 spinal nerve roots (and dorsal root ganglion) uniting to form C8 nerve.

114 A   Completely round facet extending well back on to the pedicle and well below the upper border of the body.
B   Lateral tubercle replacing the usual transverse process.
C   Inferior articular facet rounded – all these are features of T12 vertebra.

115   Typical left rib, from behind.
A   Intra-articular ligament.
B   Lateral costotransverse ligament.
C   Pleura.

116   Left first rib, from above.
A   Capsule of the costotransverse joint.
B   Scalenus medius.
C   Serratus anterior.

117   Left second rib, from above.
A   Capsule of the joint of the head of the rib.
B   Superior costotransverse ligament.
C   Serratus anterior.

118 Front of the sternum.
A Sternal end of the clavicle.
B Right second costal cartilage.
C Left fourth costal cartilage.

119 Back of the sternum.
A Sternothyroid.
B Right pleura.
C Pericardium.

120 A Left brachiocephalic vein, joining the right to form the superior vena cava.
B A thymic vein, draining to a brachiocephalic or internal thoracic vein.
C Right lobe of the thymus – from the ventral part of the right third pharyngeal pouch.

121 A Internal thoracic artery, from the first part of the subclavian – ends by dividing into the musculophrenic and superior epigastric arteries.
B Beginning of the right brachiocephalic vein – behind the sternoclavicular joint.
C Beginning of the superior vena cava – at the lower border of the first right costal cartilage.

122 A Transverse sinus, behind the ascending aorta and pulmonary trunk.
B Right coronary artery.
C An anterior cardiac vein.
D Marginal branch of the right coronary artery and the small cardiac vein.
E Anterior interventricular branch of the left coronary artery and the great cardiac vein.
F From the apex in the left fifth intercostal space about 9 cm from the midline to the left second costal cartilage at the lateral border of the sternum.

123 Interior of the right atrium, from the front.
A Smooth part of the right atrium—from the sinus venosus.
B Atrial septum in the fossa ovalis— from the septum primum (fusion with the septum secundum forms the curved margin of the fossa).
C Valve of the coronary sinus—from the lower end of the right venous valve.

124 Interior of the right ventricle, from the front.
A Anterior cusp of the tricuspid valve – a layer of fibrous tissue covered by endocardium on both sides.
B Anterior papillary muscle – from the anterolateral ventricular wall to the anterior and posterior ventricular cusps.
C Septomarginal trabecula (moderator band) – from the lower part of the interventricular septum to the base of the anterior papillary muscle.

125 Right lung root.
A Azygos vein, arching forward above the root to enter the superior vena cava.
B Right pulmonary artery, just behind the upper pulmonary vein.
C Right principal bronchus, the most posterior of the large structures in the root.

126 Left lung root.
A Left vagus nerve, passing behind the lung root after crossing the arch of the aorta.
B Left upper pulmonary vein, below the left pulmonary artery.
C Left lower lobe bronchus, here passing down behind the (cut) upper pulmonary vein.

127 Right mediastinum.
A Branch of the right pulmonary artery to the upper lobe, arising before the main artery enters the lung root.
B Right principal bronchus, the most posterior of the large structures in the lung root.
C Right lower pulmonary vein, the lowest structure in the lung root.

128 Cast of the right principal bronchus and segmental bronchi.
A Anterior bronchus of upper lobe.
B Lateral bronchus of middle lobe.
C Posterior basal bronchus of lower lobe.

129 Left mediastinum.
A Left phrenic nerve (with pericardiacophrenic vessels) crossing the arch of the aorta anterior to the vagus nerve.
B Left superior intercostal vein crossing the arch of the aorta transversely.
C Left pulmonary artery, the highest structure in the lung root.

130 A Inferior lingular bronchus of upper lobe.
B Apical (superior) bronchus of lower lobe.
C Lateral basal bronchus of lower lobe.

131 A Anterior layer of rectus sheath – aponeuroses of external and internal oblique muscles.
B Posterior layer of rectus sheath – aponeuroses of internal oblique and transversus muscles.
C Rectus abdominis – by the lower six thoracic nerves.

132 A External oblique – by the lower six thoracic nerves by their lateral cutaneous branches.
B and C Internal oblique and transversus – by the lower six thoracic nerves and by the first lumbar nerve (iliohypogastric and ilio-inguinal).

133 A T7 nerve running parallel to the costal margin.
B T8 nerve running almost horizontally (although a branch not shown here runs upwards near T7).
C T9 nerve passing obliquely downwards.

134 A At this level the borders of the two rectus muscles should lie close together.
B Transversalis fascia, extraperitoneal tissue and peritoneum.
C Inferior epigastric artery, from the external iliac, passing upwards medial to the deep inguinal ring.

135 A Deep inguinal ring – in the transversalis fascia midway between the pubic symphysis and the anterior superior iliac spine.
B Inguinal triangle – bounded by the inferior epigastric vessels, inguinal ligament and the lateral border of rectus abdominis.
C Femoral ring – bounded by the inguinal ligament, lacunar ligament, pectineus and the femoral vein.

136 A Falciform ligament – from the ventral mesogastrium.
B Ligamentum teres, the obliterated remains of the left umbilical vein.
C Fundus of the gall bladder – where the lateral border of the right rectus sheath meets the ninth costal cartilage.

137 A Lesser omentum – from the ventral mesogastrium.
B Bile duct on the right of the hepatic artery, both in front of the portal vein.
C Epiploic foramen – above, caudate process of the liver; below, first part of the duodenum; in front, portal vein; behind, inferior vena cava.

138 A Splenic artery giving pancreatic, splenic, left gastro-epiploic and short gastric branches.
B Gastroduodenal artery, giving superior pancreaticoduodenal. right gastroepiploic and pancreatic branches (and perhaps the right gastric).
C Lower end of the oesophagus – veins draining to the left gastric vein and hence to the portal system.

139 A Uncinate process of the pancreas, from the ventral pancreatic bud.
B Body of the pancreas, from the dorsal pancreatic bud.
C Middle colic branch of the superior mesenteric artery – between the two layers of the transverse mesocolon.

140 A Prepyloric vein – overlying the upper anterior part of the pylorus.
B Pyloric antrum – mucous surface cells, mucous neck cells, pyloric gland cells, G (endocrine, gastrin-secreting) cells.
C Right gastric artery – anastomosing with the left gastric along the lesser curvature.

141 Transverse section at the level of L2 vertebra.
A Bile duct, lying in a groove on the back of the pancreas medial to the descending part of the duodenum and in front of the inferior vena cava.
B Right sympathetic trunk, overlapped by the inferior vena cava.
C Superior mesenteric vein, on the right side of the artery and crossing the uncinate process of the pancreas.

142 A Right ureter, crossed by the gonadal vessels which are unusually high in this specimen.
B Descending (second) part of the duodenum, being mobilised to the left after cutting the peritoneum at its right margin.
C Inferior vena cava, becoming displaced as the duodenum is turned medially, with the right gonadal artery crossing the vein and the gonadal vein entering it.

143 Descending (second) part of the duodenum, opened from the front.
A Minor duodenal papilla, with the opening of the accessory pancreatic duct.
B Major duodenal papilla, with the opening of the hepatopancreatic ampulla which receives the bile and main pancreatic ducts.
C Inferior pancreaticoduodenal artery, from the superior mesenteric.

144 A A pancreatic vein, draining to the superior mesenteric.
B Jejunal and ileal veins, draining to the superior mesenteric.
C Jejunal and ileal branches of the superior mesenteric artery.

145 A Left genitofemoral nerve, emerging from the anterior surface of psoas major.
B Inferior mesenteric vein, lying lateral to the artery, receiving left colic tributaries and draining to the splenic vein behind the pancreas.
C Ureter, here being crossed by the gonadal vessels and the left colic artery.
(Note that the gonadal artery has arisen from the left renal artery and not from the aorta.)

146 A Fissure for the ligamentum venosum – has part of the lesser omentum attached.
B Caudate process – upper boundary of the epiploic foramen.
C Inferior layer of the coronary ligament – reflected on to the right kidney and forming the upper boundary of the hepatorenal pouch.

147 Visceral surface of the spleen.
A Left kidney.
B Stomach.
C Lienorenal ligament – containing the splenic vessels and tail of the pancreas.

148 A Common hepatic duct – formed by union of the right and left hepatic ducts.
B Bile duct – formed by union of the common hepatic and cystic ducts.
C Cystic artery – usually from the right branch of the hepatic, but may arise from the left branch of the hepatic, the hepatic itself or the gastroduodenal.

149 Transverse section of the left upper abdomen.
A Left suprarenal gland – by branches from the aorta and the left inferior phrenic and renal arteries.
B Lienorenal ligament – from the dorsal mesogastrium.
C Gastrosplenic ligament – containing the short gastric and left gastroepiploic vessels.

150 A Left gastric artery – supplying the stomach and lower part of oesophagus.
B Left suprarenal vein – draining the gland and here receiving the left inferior phrenic vein.
C Left suprarenal gland – normally covered by peritoneum of the posterior wall of the lesser sac.

151 A Lesser omentum, emerging from the porta hepatis to pass to the lesser curvature of the stomach.
B Portal vein, entering the porta hepatis behind the hepatic artery.
C Left renal vein, crossing in front of the aorta to enter the inferior vena cava.

152 A Renal capsule, adhering to the surface of the kidney.
B Renal fascia, outside the perirenal fat (scanty in this specimen).
C Anterior layer of the lumbar part of the thoracolumbar fascia, in front of quadratus lumborum.

153 A Hilum of the left kidney – 5 cm from the midline just above the transpyloric plane.
B Ureter – from the above point along a line towards the pubic tubercle.
C Ilio-inguinal nerve – skin of the inguinal region and anterior part of the scrotum (or labia).

154 A Ileocolic artery, from the superior mesenteric.
B Appendicular artery, usually from the posterior caecal branch of the ileocolic.
C Base of the appendix – McBurney's point, one third of the way along a line from the anterior superior iliac spine to the umbilicus.

155 A Posterior layer of the greater omentum (transverse colon turned upwards).
B Posterior layer of the transverse mesocolon.
C Middle colic artery, from the superior mesenteric.

156 A Ureter, after being crossed by the left colic artery, with the inferior mesenteric vein crossing the artery.
B Sigmoid branches of the inferior mesenteric artery, here arising by a common trunk with the left colic artery.
C Superior rectal artery, the continuation of the inferior mesenteric into the pelvis.

157 A Abnormal obturator artery, arising from the inferior epigastric.
B Lacunar ligament, forming the medial boundary of the femoral ring; it may have to be cut to relieve a femoral hernia.
C Ductus (vas) deferens has its own artery, a branch of the superior vesical.

158 A Conjoint tendon, formed by the lowest (aponeurotic) fibres of the internal oblique and transversus muscles.
B Spermatic cord, here covered by the cremasteric and internal spermatic fasciae.
C Spermatic cord, here covered by the external spermatic, cremasteric and internal spermatic fasciae.

159 A Head of the epididymis – from the mesonephric duct.
B Appendix of the testis – from the paramesonephric duct.
C Ductus (vas) deferens – from the mesonephric duct.

160 A Ductus (vas) deferens, crossing superficial to the ureter.
B Middle lobe of the prostate, between the urethra in front and the ejaculatory ducts behind (one duct is seen sectioned here).
C Rectovesical pouch of peritoneum, the lowest part of the peritoneal cavity and palpable on rectal examination.
D Prostate – to iliac and sacral nodes.
E Rectum – to iliac and inferior mesenteric nodes.
F Lower anal canal – to superficial inguinal nodes.

161 A Suspensory ligament of the ovary, containing the ovarian vessels.
B Mesovarium, connecting the ovary to the posterior layer of the broad ligament.
C Mesosalpinx, containing the uterine tube at the upper edge of the broad ligament.

162 A Uterus – from the paramesonephric ducts.
B Vagina – from the paramesonephric ducts.
C Urethra – from the vesico-urethral part of the urogenital sinus, which is from the front part of the cloaca.

163 A Medial limb of the sigmoid mesocolon, passing downwards and medially to the third piece of the sacrum.
B Ureter, crossing the external iliac vessels and running down in front of the internal iliac artery after passing deep to the apex of the sigmoid mesocolon.
C External iliac vein, lying medial to the artery.
D Ovary – to paraaortic and superficial inguinal nodes, and to the opposite ovary.
E Body of the uterus – to iliac, paraaortic and superficial inguinal nodes.
F Cervix of the uterus – to iliac and sacral nodes (but *not* to inguinal nodes).

164 A Ovarian vessels passing to the ovary in the suspensory ligament (here removed).
B Ligament of the ovary, connecting the uterine end of the ovary to the lateral border of the uterus behind the tube.
C Condensed retroperitoneal tissue forming the uterosacral ligament, passing from the vaginal fornix and cervix to the sacrum.

165 A Uterine artery, here crossing the ureter.
B Condensed retroperitoneal tissue lateral to the vaginal fornix and cervix, forming the lateral cervical (Mackenrodt's) ligament.
C Obturator nerve, entering the obturator foramen above the artery and vein.

166 A Tensor fasciae latae – superior gluteal nerve.
B Gluteus minimus – superior gluteal nerve.
C Straight head of rectus femoris – femoral nerve.

167 A Transverse ligament, bridging the acetabular notch.
B Adductor brevis – anterior division of the obturator nerve.
C Adductor longus – anterior division of the obturator nerve.

168 A Pectineal ligament.
B Lacunar ligament.
C Inguinal ligament.

169 A Semitendinosus and the long head of biceps – tibial part of the sciatic nerve.
B Semimembranosus – tibial part of the sciatic nerve.
C Adductor magnus – tibial part of the sciatic nerve and the posterior division of the obturator nerve.

170 A Parts of the capsule and iliofemoral ligament.
B Vastus lateralis – femoral nerve.
C Vastus intermedius – femoral nerve.

171 A Obturator externus – posterior division of the obturator nerve.
B Part of the capsule.
C Psoas major – first three lumbar nerves.

172 A Medial head of gastrocnemius – tibial nerve.
B Part of the capsule.
C Anterior cruciate ligament.

173 A Lateral head of gastrocnemius – tibial nerve.
B Fibular collateral ligament (lateral ligament).
C Popliteus – tibial nerve.

174 A Iliotibial tract – helps to stabilise the knee in full extension.
B Tendons of sartorius, gracilis and semitendinosus, all helping to flex the knee.
C Tibialis anterior – dorsiflexion and inversion of the foot.

175 A Posterior cruciate ligament.
B Anterior horn of the lateral meniscus.
C Anterior horn of the medial meniscus.

176 A Biceps – tibial part (long head) and common peroneal part (short head) of sciatic nerve.
B Semimembranosus – tibial part of sciatic nerve.
C Soleus – tibial nerve.

177 A Tendon of peroneus brevis.
B Tendon of flexor hallucis longus.
C Tendon of tibialis posterior.

178 A Extensor digitorum brevis – deep peroneal nerve.
B Peroneus brevis – superficial peroneal nerve.
C Abductor hallucis – medial plantar nerve.
D First dorsal interosseous – deep branch of the lateral plantar nerve.
E and F Tibialis anterior – deep peroneal nerve.

179 A Flexor hallucis brevis and abductor hallucis – medial plantar nerve.
B Peroneus longus – superficial peroneal nerve.
C Tibialis posterior – tibial nerve.
D Plantar calcaneonavicular ligament (spring ligament).
E Long plantar ligament.
F Flexor accessorius – lateral plantar nerve.

180 Left talus, medial side.
A Medial malleolus of tibia.
B Navicular bone.
C Plantar calcaneonavicular ligament (spring ligament).

181 Left calcaneus, upper surface.
A Part of the medial (deltoid) ligament.
B Interosseous ligament.
C Cervical ligament.

182 Left calcaneus, lateral side.
A Inferior peroneal retinaculum.
B Calcaneofibular ligament.
C Tendo calcaneus (Achilles tendon).

183 A Gluteus medius – superior gluteal nerve. Abductor of the hip but more important as a preventer of adduction when the opposite leg is off the ground as in walking.
B Common peroneal part of the sciatic nerve – L4,5, S1,2.
C Inferior gluteal artery – a terminal branch of the anterior division of the internal iliac.

184 A Anastomotic branch between the inferior gluteal and medial circumflex femoral artery, part of the cruciate anastomosis.
B Membranous upper end of semimembranosus, overlying adductor magnus.
C Nerve to the short head of biceps – the only branch to arise from the lateral side of the sciatic nerve (common peroneal part).

185 A Medial circumflex femoral artery – from the profunda femoris but often directly from the femoral.
B Obturator externus – posterior division of the obturator nerve.
C Adductor brevis – anterior division of the obturator nerve.

186 A Femoral artery – behind it the tendon of psoas major crossing the middle of the hip joint capsule.
B Femoral nerve – behind it iliacus joining the lateral side of the psoas tendon.
C Nerve to adductor longus – between the branches to adductor brevis and gracilis, all lying on adductor brevis between pectineus above and adductor longus below.

187 A Sartorius, displaced laterally over rectus femoris to reveal nerve and vessel branches.
B Transverse branch of the lateral femoral circumflex artery, passing deep to rectus femoris.
C Saphenous nerve, passing down on the medial side of the femoral artery in front of the nerve to vastus medialis.

188 Coronal section of the left hip, from the front.
A Acetabular labrum, of fibrocartilage, attached to the rim of the acetabulum and below becoming continuous with the transverse ligament.
B Gluteus medius – to the lateral side of the greater trochanter.
C Psoas major – to the lesser trochanter.

189 A Upper margin of the saphenous opening, overlapping the femoral vein.
B Superficial epigastric vein.
C Superficial circumflex iliac vein. Both join the great saphenous vein (in this specimen by a common trunk with an anterolateral vein).

190 Cross section of the right upper thigh, from below.
A Femoral artery with the vein on the lateral side, sartorius medially, vastus medialis in front and adductor magnus behind.
B Gracilis with the great saphenous vein medially.
C Semimembranosus with semitendinosus laterally.

191 Right knee, lateral side.
A Iliotibial tract; the groove (shadow) below it is due to the attachment of the fascia lata to the lateral intermuscular septum.
B Biceps tendon passing forwards to the head of the fibula.
C Tibial tuberosity receiving the patellar ligament.

192 A Common peroneal nerve, lying medial to the tendon of biceps.
B Sural nerve, a branch of the tibial nerve and lying adjacent to the small saphenous vein.
C Tendon of semitendinosus lying on semimembranosus which is wider.

193 A Bursa (which sometimes communicates with the knee joint) under the medial head of gastrocnemius.
B Plantaris, here fused with the lateral head of gastrocnemius which arises from the lateral *side* of the femur, not from the popliteal surface.
C Oblique popliteal ligament, from the tendon of semimembranosus and reinforcing the posterior surface of the capsule.

194 A Fibular collateral ligament (lateral ligament), passing from the lateral epicondyle of the femur to the head of the fibula.
B Medial meniscus, connected to the tibial collateral ligament (medial ligament).
C Posterior meniscofemoral ligament, joining the posterior part of the lateral meniscus to the lateral side of the medial condyle and overlying the posterior cruciate ligament.

195 A Sartorius, displaced backwards (with the overlying great saphenous vein, saphenous nerve and its infrapatellar branch) to show the popliteal fossa from the medial side.
B Popliteal artery, the deepest of the neurovascular structures in the fossa.
C Tendon of adductor magnus attached to the adductor pubercle.

196 Cross section of the left upper leg, from below.
A Extensor digitorum longus, superficial to extensor hallucis longus with tibialis anterior medially.
B Peroneus longus overlying peroneus brevis.
C Tibial nerve, with tibialis posterior in front and soleus behind, and large adjacent veins.

197 A A branch to tibialis anterior from the deep peroneal nerve.
B Deep peroneal nerve – supplying tibialis anterior, extensor hallucis longus, extensor digitorum longus, peroneus tertius and extensor digitorum brevis.
C Superficial peroneal nerve – supplying peroneus longus and brevis.

198 A Anterior tibial artery – becomes the dorsalis pedis artery on crossing the ankle joint.
B Deep peroneal nerve – medial terminal branch supplying skin of the first toe cleft, and lateral terminal branch supplying extensor digitorum brevis and interosseous branches.
C Extensor digitorum longus – forms tendons for the second to fifth toes.

199 A Synovial sheath of tibialis anterior, extending above the upper margin of the superior extensor retinaculum.
B Upper limb of the inferior extensor retinaculum, passing to the medial malleolus.
C Synovial sheath of extensor hallucis longus, extending above the inferior retinaculum but not under the superior.

200 A Tendon of extensor digitorum brevis to the great toe, sometimes called extensor hallucis brevis, lying medial to extensor hallucis longus.
B Deep plantar branch of the first dorsal metatarsal artery, passing into the sole between the heads of the first dorsal interosseous muscle.
C Tendon of extensor digitorum longus to the third toe, here overlying the tendon of extensor digitorum brevis to the second toe.

201 A Tibialis posterior – plantarflexion and inversion of the foot.
B Flexor digitorum longus – plantarflexion of the foot and flexion of the second to fifth toes.
C Tendo calcaneus (Achilles tendon, for gastrocnemius and soleus) – plantarflexion of the foot.

202 A Peroneus longus – to the medial side of the medial cuneiform and the base of the first metatarsal.
B Peroneus brevis – to the tuberosity of the base of the fifth metatarsal.
C Peroneus tertius – variable, to the base and/or shaft of the fifth metatarsal.

203 A Lateral branch of the superficial peroneal nerve – supplying skin of the third and fourth toe clefts.
B Perforating branch from the peroneal artery.
C Lateral malleolar branch from the anterior tibial artery.

204 A Posterior articular surface of the calcaneus – articulating with the posterior articular surface of the talus.
B Cartilage on the upper surface of the plantar calcaneonavicular (spring) ligament – articulating with the under surface of the head of the talus.
C Posterior surface of the navicular – articulating with the front of the head of the talus.

205 Right ankle, from the right and behind.

A Tendo calcaneus (Achilles tendon) – on the middle facet of the posterior surface of the calcaneus.

B Small saphenous vein – pierces the deep fascia over the popliteal fossa to enter the popliteal vein.

C Sural nerve – continues on to the lateral side of the foot and little toe.

206 Right ankle, from the medial side.

A Saphenous nerve – on the medial side of the foot as far forward as the metatarsophalangeal joint of the great toe.

B Great saphenous vein – joins the femoral vein at the saphenous opening, 3.5 cm below and lateral to the pubic tubercle.

C Medial calcanean branch of the tibial nerve – skin of the heel and medial side of the sole.

207 A First common plantar digital nerve (from the medial plantar) – first lumbrical and skin of the first cleft.

B Fourth common plantar digital nerve (from the lateral plantar) – skin of the fourth cleft.

C Deep branch of the lateral plantar nerve – to all lumbricals except the first, all interossei except the third plantar and fourth dorsal, and adductor hallucis.

208 A Tendon of peroneus longus lying in its groove on the under surface of the cuboid and displayed by removal of the overlying part of the long plantar ligament.

B Plantar calcaneocuboid ligament (short plantar ligament), partly under cover of the long plantar.

C Main insertion of tibialis posterior, into the tuberosity of the navicular.

Index